"Chris Freytag shares an easy process to turn things you do every day without thinking (these are called habits) into your very own highly effective fitness routines. By making only slight changes in your current habits, you create new, positive habits that help you become healthier, more energetic, and more confident."

—Larry Wilson, author of *Play to Win: Choosing Growth Over Fear in Work and Life*

"Solid advice for anyone who wants to be lean and strong...for life. Chris Freytag motivates, educates, and provides simple, medically sound, easy-to-follow programs that will transform your body."

—Nicholas A. DiNubile, MD, author of *FrameWork: Your 7-Step Program for Healthy Muscles, Bones, and Joints;* orthopedic consultant, Philadelphia 76ers and the Pennsylvania Ballet

"Chris Freytag has assembed an extraordinary resource for a practical personal program for weight loss that is based on sound research from the exercise and nutrition sciences. All who adhere to a plan incorporating the great variety of exercises, the principles for exercising, and the nutrition information included can maintain their most appropriate body weight and will be more physically fit."

—Ash Hayes, EdD, ACSM emeritus; former executive director, President's Council on Physical Fitness and Sports; and board member, American Council on Exercise

"Chris Freytag's book *Prevention's Shortcuts to Big Weight Loss* does an excellent job translating current research findings in exercise science and human nutrition into an easy-to-understand and compassionate guide to physical activity and healthy eating that will resonate with most readers. This book works as well for the committed jock as it does for the couch potato. Ms. Freytag identifies simple but effective strategies to help people change their behavior and combine sensible physical activity with realistic nutritional goals."

—Wojtek J. Chodzko-Zajko, PhD, professor and head of the department of kinesiology and community health, University of Illinois at Urbana-Champaign

"This book strips away all of the nonsense and pseudoscience usually associated with weight loss programs, so all that's left is what really works. It's a must-read for anyone who is serious about losing weight and keeping it off."

—Liz Neporent, author of *The Fat-Free Truth and Fitness for Dummies*

Prevention's
SHORTCUTS TO
BIG
WEIGHT
LOSS

**SLIM YOUR BELLY, BUTT, AND THIGHS—
AND GET FIT TWICE AS FAST**

CHRIS FREYTAG

RODALE

Notice

The information in this book is meant to supplement, not replace, proper exercise training. All forms of exercise pose some inherent risks. The editors and publisher advise readers to take full responsibility for their safety and know their limits. Before practicing the exercises in this book, be sure that your equipment is well-maintained, and do not take risks beyond your level of experience, aptitude, training, and fitness. The exercise and dietary programs in this book are not intended as a substitute for any exercise routine or dietary regimen that may have been prescribed by your doctor. As with all exercise and dietary programs, you should get your doctor's approval before beginning.

Mention of specific companies, organizations, or authorities in this book does not imply endorsement by the author or publisher, nor does mention of specific companies, organizations, or authorities imply that they endorse this book, its author, or the publisher.

Internet addresses and telephone numbers given in this book were accurate at the time it went to press.

Recipes in this book have previously appeared in *Prevention* magazine.

Direct edition first published in 2007. Trade edition published in 2008.

© 2007 by Motivating Bodies, Inc.
Photographs © 2007 by Rodale Inc.

Rodale books may be purchased for business or promotional use or for special sales. For information, please write to: Special Markets Department, Rodale Inc., 733 Third Avenue, New York, NY 10017

Prevention is a registered trademark of Rodale Inc.
Printed in the United States of America

Rodale Inc. makes every effort to use acid-free ⊗, recycled paper ♻.

Photographs by Mitch Mandel/Rodale Images
Book design by Christina Gaugler

Library of Congress Cataloging-in-Publication Data

Freytag, Chris.
Prevention's shortcuts to big weight loss : slim your belly, butt, and thighs—and get fit twice as fast / Chris Freytag.
     p.   cm.
     Includes index.
     ISBN-13 978–1–59486–541–1 hardcover
     ISBN-10 1–59486–541–8 hardcover
     ISBN-13 978–1–59486–540–4 paperback
     ISBN-10 1–59486–540–X paperback
     1. Reducing exercises.   2. Weight loss.   3. Abdominal exercises.   I. Title.
     RA781.6.F74   2007
     613.7—dc22   2007007159

Distributed to the trade by Macmillan

2   4   6   8   10   9   7   5   3   1   hardcover
2   4   6   8   10   9   7   5   3   1   paperback

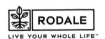

LIVE YOUR WHOLE LIFE™

We inspire and enable people to improve their lives and the world around them
For more of our products visit **rodalestore.com** or call 1-800-848-4735

Contents

Acknowledgments

A book is a labor of love. There are so many people to thank who helped me along the way.

First, a big thanks to my family, who live, breathe, and eat fitness with me every day. I appreciate all the patience and support during the long hours and nutty deadlines.

To Selene Yeager, my cowriter and friend, thanks for all your hard work. Your eloquence is much appreciated!

To my editor, Kathy LeSage, for your advice and guidance. Your knowledge and expertise helped form this book.

A huge thanks to all the others at Rodale who made this book happen. I feel lucky to work with you all.

And, of course, to all of my clients, viewers, and dear friends—you inspire me each and every day.

Foreword

Chris Freytag has been a good friend of mine for more than 20 years. I've also had the opportunity to work with her in the business world over the past 7 years. As a working mother and fitness enthusiast myself, I've been fortunate to benefit from Chris's passion for helping others live better lives by making healthy lifestyle changes.

On a personal level, Chris was my motivator to break through barriers and run my first 10-mile race. She not only coached me but ran the race with me. That's the kind of person she is—with you right to the end.

On a business level, I've also had the chance to see Chris motivate and coach. As a former senior vice president for a major department store, I consulted Chris to help the retail chain institute a fitness department in each of their stores. Her knowledge of the needs of the customers and her ability to direct the product contributed to instant success. As the former executive vice president of ShopNBC, I worked directly with Chris as she developed a fitness business from nothing for the home shopping channel. Chris helped the network build an assortment of fitness-related products and accessories. Her ability to relate to people, wherever they are on their health and fitness journeys, created tremendous success for the network, as evidenced by the fantastic sales and the thousands of e-mails Chris received.

Chris is always listening to the needs of people around her. She understands how busy people's lives are, and, as you will see in this book, she recommends a realistic approach to get you where you want to be. I have watched so many women pour out their hearts to Chris, sharing their unique challenges and the results they were able to achieve, thanks to her advice about diet and exercise. She has her finger on the pulse of American habits and is constantly suggesting ways to live a more balanced and fit life. You won't find a more authentic fitness expert.

Chris's advice is safe and easy to understand—and it works. She always tells her clients that there is no magic pill for weight loss. But this book is the closest thing out there. After reading it, you will be more educated and more motivated. You will have a realistic plan that fits your busy lifestyle. And you will get what we are all looking for: better results.

Liz Haesler
Vice President, Best Buy Corporation

PART 1

Speed Your Way to Weight Loss with *Prevention's* Shortcuts

CHAPTER 1

Shorter Is Better

"I'm too busy to work out!"

"It's all I can do to shower and get dressed! When am I going to exercise?"

Those are the laments I hear every day from overscheduled, stressed-out women around the country: women who think that unless they go to the gym for hours a day, they'll never lose weight; who think that exercise must be arduous and time-consuming for it to count.

That mind-set isn't only misguided, it's making us fat.

Consider two typical busy modern women. One desperately tries to make it to step aerobics class 3 days a week but is otherwise chained to her desk or stuck in her car. The other never steps foot in the gym but takes two or three 10-minute walks a day and performs a few easy dumbbell exercises in the evening. Who do you think gets fitter faster?

You might be surprised to learn that the fitter woman is the second one, by a long shot. She stays saner and happier, too!

Long before there were gyms, health clubs, and celebrity trainers, people didn't carve out 60 minutes to climb flight after flight of steps on a StairMaster. They got fit and *stayed* fit 1 minute at a time just by moving their bodies. And that's the only way we're going to turn our crazy, busy, yet all-too-sedentary lives into crazy, busy, *active* lives. I'm going to show you *exactly* how, with a totally fresh—yet amazingly commonsense—approach to fitness: *Prevention's Shortcuts to Big Weight Loss.*

Prevention's Shortcuts are workouts that I've specially designed to give you the maximum fat-burning, body-toning power possible in just 10 minutes. But this program isn't just about convenience. *Prevention's* Shortcuts deliver better results in less time than the traditional 30- to 40-minute workout approach that has been drilled into our heads. That's right, my 10-minute *Prevention's* Shortcuts workouts actually work *better* than longer exercise sessions. I see it with the hundreds of women I train—and it's 100 percent scientifically proven.

By committing yourself to *Prevention's Shortcuts to Big Weight Loss*, I promise you can

- Drop up to two dress sizes in 8 weeks.

- Lose 30 percent more weight with these 10-minute workouts than with 40-minute walking workouts.

- Burn an extra 200 calories a day. (That means you'll be zapping the equivalent of a pack of M&M'S every single day.)

- Increase your cardiovascular fitness more than *twice* as quickly as you would doing traditional 30- to 40-minute workouts.

- Reduce your heart disease risk and key risk factors like triglycerides, dropping them lower and faster than you would by following a more traditional workout system.

- Maybe most important, you'll *keep* your weight off better, too!

And that's not all! You'll have more energy, feel happier, build strong bones, improve your posture, and—here's the best part—still have time for your family, friends, and everything else in your life that you love.

THE SECRET OF MY OWN SUCCESS

Hi. I'm Chris Freytag, and I live your life. I'm not a rich celebrity with a live-in trainer, chef, and personal assistant. I'm a working mother of three from Minnesota. I'm emptying the dishwasher, folding laundry, driving carpools, and correcting homework just like you. I'm over 40, and I'm a realist. I know that as we age, our obligations become more time-consuming, and spending time with those we care about gets harder to do. So free time is more precious than gold. I know that all those crazy post-35 hormone changes can make your hips widen and waistline expand, even if you're eating less. I know that as time passes, there are more chances for health issues to surface. But here's what else I know: Once you acknowledge your life—cherish it for all its beauty and goodness—and take charge of the life you're living, instead of hoping it somehow changes on its own (or worse, trying to live someone else's life), *that's* when the really good stuff happens. That's when you get fit, lose weight, and look and feel great.

Like you (unless you're *really* enlightened), I wasn't as concerned with any of this stuff 20 years ago, even though I was already in the fitness industry. I breezed through my twenties, eating desserts, enjoying after-work wine with friends, and never worrying about my weight. But my body started to change in my thirties. I had three kids, and I noticed the toll it took on my time, emotions, and appearance. It forced me to take a more active role in my health.

Now that I'm in my forties, I feel like I'm in the best shape of my life, mentally, spiritually, and physically. Everyone always asks, "What's your secret?" I practice what I preach! I do longer workouts when I can, because I love to move my body. But when I have less time on my hands (as is so often the case these days), I just seize every opportunity to squeeze in a little *Prevention*'s Shortcuts activity. I'll do *Prevention*'s Shortcuts core-strengthening moves, featured in Chapter 8, while watching the news. If I'm traveling, I'll do Chapter 12's yoga workouts in my hotel room. Some days, all I can manage is one of Chapter 4's cardio walking workouts on the treadmill. But I do it. *And it works.*

That is the heart and soul of the *Prevention's Shortcuts to Big Weight Loss* program. It's a program that gets you fit on your own time, working with your specific limitations and needs. So it fits seamlessly into your life whether you're a stay-at-home mother of four or a working single woman who's a desk jockey. I've seen it transform hundreds of women's lives. Now it can transform yours. You'll learn how to identify workout opportunities—I call them Shortcut Slots—you never knew existed. And I'll tell you *exactly* what moves to do to make the most of those free moments. You'll find 48 safe, efficient, 10-minute workouts you can do every day without missing a beat— or your book club meeting!

LOSE FAT, KEEP IT OFF, AND MORE

I can hear you now. You're thinking, "No way will I ever lose these saddlebags or tighten this tummy with a 10-minute workout. Everything I read says I need at least 30 minutes of exercise." Well, here's the thing: No one ever said you had to do all 30 of those minutes at one time! In fact, there's very compelling scientific evidence that spreading out activity over the course of the day may not only be easier to do, but may also work faster and be better for you, too.

Over the past few years, numerous studies have shown that women can lose weight, lower their heart disease risk, and improve their aerobic fitness by adopting the *Prevention*'s Shortcuts approach to exercise. Without bogging you down with science, here are a few standouts.

Fat loss. In a 20-week study of 56 overweight, sedentary women, researchers at the University of Pittsburgh found that those who were advised to perform multiple 10-minute bouts of exercise throughout the day were better able to stick to the program and lost more weight than those who had been told to get their exercise in one 30- to 40-minute chunk three times a week. Specifically, the short-bouters worked out an average of 4 days a week, versus 3 days for the long-bout group; they were active about 32 minutes a day, versus 27 minutes for the long-bouters; and by the end of the study, they shed an average of 20 pounds, 6 more than those who tried to squeeze in all their exercise in one shot. That's 30 percent more weight loss from short bouts of exercise like *Prevention*'s Shortcuts than from a traditional exercise program. One woman in the study even lost more than 30 pounds!

10-SECOND WISDOM
"Work out smarter, not longer."

In a similar study from Singapore, researchers divided a group of 30 overweight women into two groups. Twice a week, one group walked or cycled on exercise machines until they burned 1,000 calories. The other worked out 5 days a week, on the same machines, burning 400 calories each time. None of the women changed what they ate. After 8 weeks, both groups had lost nearly identical amounts of weight, body fat, and inches off their waists.

Some researchers theorize that multiple short bursts of activity burn fat as well as, if not better than, a single long bout because they keep your metabolism revved throughout the day. Your calorie burn stays elevated for up to an hour after you finish exercising. So you get more total after-exercise calorie burn throughout the day with several *Prevention*'s Shortcuts than you do with one long workout. That means you actually burn more calories for the same total exercise time.

Heart health. Physical activity is like a Roto-Rooter for your arteries, flushing them clean and keeping them clear and supple. A study published in *Medicine & Science in Sports & Exercise* found that accumulated 10-minute bursts of exercise (like *Prevention*'s Shortcuts) throughout the day were actually more effective at lowering triglycerides—a type of blood fat that raises your heart attack risk—than one continuous 30-minute jog on the treadmill. Why? Because, like I mentioned above, short bouts have a more positive effect on metabolism, so your body burns more fat, including the fat floating through your bloodstream, all day long. Thomas Altena, EdD, the author of this study, was quoted as saying, "People who cannot exercise for long durations due to low fitness levels or busy lifestyles don't have to sit still and wait for a heart attack." I couldn't agree more! A strong, healthy heart is just one more reason why I recommend you do at least three *Prevention*'s Shortcuts a day.

Cardio fitness. Challenging your body with a few high-energy bouts of exercise—like 30- to 120-second fast-paced intervals on a treadmill or stationary bike—can improve your endurance as much as slogging along at a slower pace for hours each week. In one Canadian study, researchers found that men and women who cranked out four 30-second sprints (with 4 minutes of rest between efforts) on exercise bikes three times a week reaped fitness gains identical to those who pedaled for *2 hours* at a moderate pace three times a week! I love this approach, because it's much easier to psych yourself into doing something—even if it's a little hard—for just 30 seconds or a minute or two than it is to rally your energy for an hour-long haul. The Quick Calorie Burners, Fat-Sizzling Walking Workouts, and Bun Burners in Chapter 4 are great interval workouts for building cardiovascular fitness.

Furthermore, the *Prevention*'s Shortcuts program may improve your cardio health twice as quickly as other programs. In another study, University of New Hampshire researchers asked 37 men and women to perform either two short-bout workouts (15 minutes each) or one continuous 30-minute exercise bout 4 days a week for 12 weeks. Though both groups enjoyed improved fitness, short bouts consistently worked better. The short-bouters boosted their maximal oxygen consumption (a measure of how strong their heart, lungs, and muscles became) by 8.7 percent—

nearly twice as much as the increase in the 30-minute exercisers (who improved just 4.5 percent). Short-bout exercisers also improved the amount of time they could go full out on a treadmill test by more than a minute (71 seconds), compared with a 41-second improvement in their peers doing longer bouts. Finally, only short-bout exercises raised levels of healthy HDL cholesterol. On *Prevention*'s Shortcuts plan, you'll do two short cardio workouts 3 to 5 days a week instead of conventional, longer aerobic workouts.

Sustained weight loss. How many people do you know who go on an "exercise kick," drop a bunch of weight, burn out, and gain it all back? They do this because their programs aren't sustainable. It's common sense: If exercise is easy to stick to, your results will stick, too. Research proves it. In a 2-year study of more than 230 overweight and inactive men and women, researchers at the Cooper Institute for Aerobics Research in Dallas found that those who sneaked 30 minutes of activity into their day by taking the stairs at the office, walking around the field during their kids' soccer practice, or pulling weeds around the yard shed as much body fat (and improved their fitness and heart health) as those who went to the gym to vigorously exercise for 20 to 60 minutes, 5 days a week. A Johns Hopkins University study echoed these findings, reporting that people who added just 30 minutes of lifestyle activity to their day lost almost 10 pounds during a 16-week study period—*more* than a comparable group that did step aerobics 3 days a week. What's more, the life-style exercisers did a better job of keeping the weight off.

So in addition to the 10-minute *Prevention*'s Shortcuts workouts that I've specially designed to be convenient, quick, and addictive, throughout the book you'll find Lifestyle Shortcuts, ways to make fat-burning activity a natural part of your life. You'll also learn 1-Minute Wonder workouts, 60 seconds of exercise that burns 10 extra calories—an effort that, made daily, can add up to an extra pound of weight loss each year. And in Chapter 3, we'll help you identify Shortcut Slots, the gaps in your busy schedule that can be filled with all this weight-maintaining movement.

Muscle tone. It hasn't been extensively studied, but you don't need expensive research to tell you that your butt won't get any less toned if you work it on a different day than your biceps. Breaking up your strength training routine beats the boredom of spending a half hour with your dumbbells, and you're less likely to shortchange your workout by skipping sets or reps because you're running low on time. So while *Prevention*'s Shortcuts to losing 25 pounds or more, in Chapter 5, are specially designed to work your whole body in just 10 minutes, I've also included other chapters with workouts to specifically tone individual body parts. Even when your main goal is weight loss, I give you permission—encouragement, even—to peek at Part 3, *Prevention*'s Shortcuts to Shaping and Sculpting, and deviously try one of the more narrowly targeted workouts. I happen to be one of those creative, change-it-up girls. Join me—let your hair down and go wild for 10 minutes. It'll keep you interested in and compliant with the *Prevention*'s Shortcuts program, because—here comes the common sense—the bottom line is, you must comply with the program to see results.

THE PRACTICAL APPLICATION

Even more important than what science says is the fact that *Prevention*'s Shortcuts just make sense. Before "aerobics" and fancy exercise classes, people rarely "worked out," but very few people were overweight. They didn't have to block out huge chunks of time to jog 6 miles and lift weights for an hour; they were simply running around, living active lives. Even though almost every modern woman could use more exercise, for millions of us, it feels uncomfortable and downright unnatural to run, jog, or even walk for 30 minutes or an hour nonstop. But almost everyone enjoys the instant lift from a walk around the block, like the cardio walking workouts in Chapter 4, or a nice 10-minute stretch break, like the flexibility shortcuts in Chapter 12. It's easy. And it's what your body craves. So we need to put aside this mind-set of needing a grueling 2-hour workout to whip ourselves into shape.

Here's just one example of how the approach you'll learn in this book will make a dramatic difference in your weight—and fast. My client Meghan, 32, gained 60 pounds while pregnant with her daughter, now 2, and just couldn't seem to shake the 35 she still had left to lose. Making things a little more complicated was the fact that she also had three teenage stepsons. Meghan had just about thrown in the towel when I convinced her to try *Prevention*'s Shortcuts. Here's what she had to say, in her own words.

I used to think that in order for exercise to count, I had to have an hour or two of free time, which is virtually impossible with four kids in the house. When Chris encouraged me to think about the program as simply being more active, it all started to fall into place. I found ways to fit in those 10-minute workouts. I was actually enjoying it. The first couple of days I felt more tired, but then I turned a corner and had more energy. Before long, I started feeling so good that running on the treadmill didn't seem like a chore, just more activity.

It worked! I was really amazed that in just under 2 months, I lost 15 pounds. I wish I had realized years ago that a few minutes of increased activity a few times a day could have such a big impact. I have gone down almost two dress sizes and am wearing clothes I haven't worn for years.

Now I'm continuing to work on resistance training. I'd never done much of that in the past, but the more I do, the stronger I feel, the more energy I have, and the easier it is to be active. I just fit in small segments of strength training here and there. I've lost over 20 pounds so far, and it's never felt easier.

That's right, Meghan dropped two dress sizes in less than 2 months. For a step-by-step look at how Meghan fit *Prevention's* Shortcuts into her busy schedule, check out her makeover on page 46.

You, too, can experience results like Meghan's using the *Prevention's* Shortcuts workout system. The program is carefully crafted to maximize every active minute for optimum calorie burn and metabolism revving all day long. Studies prove it, but more important, women who try it see results. You'll find more *Prevention's* Shortcuts success stories throughout the book. Try the program and soon you'll have one of your own.

TIME PASSES—DON'T LET IT PASS YOU BY!

What are you waiting for? Today will pass. This month will go by. The year will come and go whether or not you decide to make the commitment to the *Prevention's* Shortcuts lifestyle. The choice is 100 percent yours. You can wake up in 30 days and be slimmer, more toned, happier, and healthier because you've finally devoted the few minutes it takes to take care of yourself. Or you can wake up with the same old worries and body woes, wondering when you're ever going to find the time to get going.

Making exercise a habit starts with a decision that you've already made by buying this book. That decision is followed by an action—doing just one of the *Prevention's Shortcuts* workouts. That action, repeated over time, becomes a habit. And that habit becomes a way of life. That's how those women you envy, who look great and always seem to find time to exercise, do it: one step at a time.

So here you go. I'm passionate about helping people move toward better mental and physical health. I believe in you, and I'm going to spend the next 350 pages getting you motivated and moving. You see, passion means that you really care about something and want to make a difference. So I ask you: How much do you really care? Deep down, we all want to be healthy. So let's do this together. Those of us who've raised kids have already learned that it's not always easy to get things right. We screw up and make mistakes, but we don't give up, because we're passionate about our children. I have gone to bed feeling defeated as a parent only to awake the next day with a new attitude and the spirit to take it all on again. I want to help you apply that same passion to yourself and your health. I'm all about reality and telling it like it is. And I'm telling you, you can do it. Don't give up. Tackle your fears, embrace your desires, and create the body you've always wanted.

10-SECOND WISDOM

"Health and fitness isn't a destination. It's a journey we travel through our whole life. There's no place we reach where we say, 'Yes! I'm done!' We just continue on and change with age and lifestyle. The way I stay in shape at 41 is different than what I did at 21. You will hit detours and delays and potholes along the way. Just steer around them and keep going. Consider this book your map. You would never take a road trip without a planned course. Treat your fitness journey the same way."

Albert Einstein once said, "Nothing happens until something moves." He was speaking of science, but he might just as well have been referring to our lives—and our bodies. Most people are imprisoned by inertia. The only way to break free is to do something. Turn the page and get started today!

CHAPTER 2

The Time Is Now

National surveys report that one-third of women does *zero* leisure-time physical activity. Another third doesn't do enough to gain any meaningful health benefits. That means two-thirds of women literally run their lives planted on their backsides. Why? The same excuses we all have. No time. No energy. No motivation. The *Prevention*'s Shortcuts approach blows all those "nos" out of the water. Find your favorite excuses in the following pages and see what I mean.

DON'T SHORTCHANGE YOURSELF WITH THESE EXCUSES

"I'm busy." If I had a dollar for every woman who tells me she doesn't have time to work out, I could afford a month at Canyon Ranch. I'm not buying those same old excuses. "Busy" has become the new "fine": "How've you been?" "Busy." *Everyone* is busy. So here's a statistic that might shock you: Studies show that Americans actually have almost 5 hours more free time per week than we did in the 1960s. That's right, we actually have *more* free time these days. It just *feels* like a whole lot less. For one, technology allows us to cram every single waking second with activity. You can write a report, order new shoes online, call a friend, download the new iTunes, and catch up on the news in less than an hour without ever leaving your chair. Americans are masters of multitasking. By chipping away at our to-do lists throughout the day, we accomplish a gargantuan amount of work.

Between work and family obligations, our free time is also more fragmented than it used to be. So instead of one unbroken chunk of time, we end up with an hour here, a half hour there, and 20 minutes between appointments. That means when you say you're too busy to work out, it may be true—*if* you're trying to find an hour to get to the gym. But *everyone* has 10 minutes here and there that they can fill with *Prevention*'s Shortcuts.

Getting fit doesn't have to be any more time-consuming than grabbing the dry cleaning or picking out a birthday card for a friend. We just think it does because we've fallen victim to what I call the "30-minute exercise myth." For years, everyone from fitness gurus to the US government has been telling us we need to be active at least 30 minutes a day to lose weight and get fit. Unfortunately, most women think that means "Go to the gym and work my butt off on the StairMaster for a half hour straight every day."

So let's say you join a gym that's 5 or 6 miles from your house. If you're like most women, here's what will inevitably happen.

Activity	Time Spent
After work, you drive to the gym.	15 minutes with traffic
You go to the locker room to change.	5–10 minutes
You stand around waiting for a free stairclimber or treadmill.	5 minutes
You work out halfheartedly because you're bored 7 minutes into the workout.	30 minutes
You head back to the locker room to shower and change.	10–15 minutes
You drive home.	15 minutes
Total time	**90 minutes**

Sound familiar? What just happened? That "simple" 30-minute workout just turned into a 1½-hour odyssey, that's what. Is it any wonder why you stick to that program for a grand total of 2 weeks (if that long) before you start making excuses and the gym becomes a distant, guilty memory?

(continued on page 16)

Prevention's Shortcuts Success Story

"I CAN SEE MYSELF STICKING WITH THIS PROGRAM FOR LIFE."

My entire adult life I have been on a roller coaster of diets, and my weight has been on a roller coaster as well. I feel like I am finally, for once, in control. The workouts started slow, a couple of times a week, and now have blossomed into at least five times a week. I am loving the feeling of wanting to get up and move to lose some weight. I am feeling great about this program. This is the last roller coaster I am going on. I am finding time in my day, instead of making excuses. The time is there—you just have to look for it!

The short workouts were what got me going. After committing to make some changes to my life and body shape, I started slow and have worked to increase my "moving" time gradually. There are times I feel tired and unmotivated, but then I think, "Ten minutes . . . just move for 10 minutes." As soon as I start, 10 minutes fly by so quickly that I think, "Okay, 10 more minutes." The next day, I start to feel muscle soreness in places where I've never felt it before. I must be doing something right, and it feels awesome!

My starting weight was 220. I would love to be able to blame that on the three babies I had or the slow metabolism that I have always said I was gypped to get in the gene pool, but I do believe that I have no one to blame but myself. The first week on the *Prevention*'s Shortcuts program, I lost more than 2 pounds. The second week, I also lost 2-plus pounds. The third week, I was up a half pound and feeling discouraged, but I kept on. Even when I went on vacation, I kept on, exercising when I could, and by the 4th week, I was down another 3-plus pounds. I began my new life venture on October 10 (a date that I will remember forever), and after 5 weeks, I had lost 11 pounds.

I have now been on the program for 6 months (wow!) and am currently down 30 pounds. I have lost 16 inches from all over.

I got myself to this weight, and I can get myself to my goal weight of 150. I can't remember the last time I weighed 150, but when it happens again, I will be celebrating! I now have the base knowledge I need and great workout routines that can fit into my crazy life's schedule.

This is a life change for me. This is forever. I really feel as though I have changed, and I look forward to the workouts. I've had my bad days, or even bad series of days, but I try not to beat myself up over them, and I get right back into the exercise (and eating) routine.

—*Stephanie, 39*

It doesn't have to be that way. It *shouldn't* be that way. Just ask obesity researcher James Levine, MD, PhD, of the Mayo Clinic: "Think back 30 years ago, before we had this obesity problem. How many people ever belonged to a gym? Nobody." People just moved more throughout the day, every day—a strategy that still works. In a fascinating study, Dr. Levine and his co-workers used revolutionary motion-monitoring underwear (there's an invention I love) to record every toe tap, fidget, and step made by 20 men and women (half lean and half obese) for 10 days. The difference between the two groups: Each day, the trim volunteers were in motion more than 2 additional hours—150 minutes—than were their overweight, completely inactive peers, despite both groups holding similarly sedentary jobs. So the slender folks burned up to 350 more calories each day. That's a pound's worth of calories every 10 days! The answer to obesity isn't more gyms, says Dr. Levine. "It's to find ways to make your life more active all day every day."

I couldn't agree more. The *Prevention's* Shortcuts program will arm you with concrete, maximally efficient routines you can do during breaks in your day to stay active and keep your metabolism revved to its full calorie-burning potential. The payoff: Every time you seize the moment to get fit, you'll feel more energized and empowered to do more.

Still think you're too busy? Starting on page 42, I'll help you examine your schedule to identify Shortcut Slots where you can squeeze in *Prevention's* Shortcuts workouts. Remember, people who are in shape and active and happy don't have more minutes in the day than you do. They've just figured out how best to use those minutes. You can learn to do that, too.

"I'm bored." Women often force themselves into activities that don't interest them or, worse, that they hate—like jogging around the block—because they think that's what they "have" to do to lose weight. Little wonder it feels like you're back in third-grade history class on a sunny spring day, wondering if time could pass any slower. You're suffering! And if you're trying to follow traditional exercise recommendations, you may be suffering for 45 minutes, which is hard for anyone to swallow. Here's my promise to you: *Prevention's* Shortcuts workouts will be so quick, easy, and fun that they'll be over and done before you have time to get bored. What's more, starting on page 19, I'll help you identify active hobbies you actually enjoy, so you'll be excited about making time for *Prevention's* Shortcuts. Now there's a revelation.

"I never see results, so why bother?" If you decide you're going to get up every morning at 5:00 a.m. and go to the gym for a half hour before work, you're going to want to see that scale move . . . and pronto! This all-too-common all-or-nothing attitude is why so many people have so little success. They try to make these big, sweeping changes, feel defeated when they haven't lost 5 pounds in 3 days, and throw in the towel. That won't happen with *Prevention*'s Shortcuts. You won't feel overwhelmed by the commitment, so you won't feel frustrated and impatient. Going back to the studies I cited earlier, you'll have an easier time fitting the *Prevention*'s Shortcuts workouts into your day, every day, so you actually will see results faster and have more motivation to keep going. I've included some of the fastest-working moves I know in Chapter 4. After just 2 weeks, you'll be sure to see results.

> **10-SECOND WISDOM**
> "If you keep doing what you're doing, you'll keep getting what you're getting."

"I'm waiting for the right time." Haven't you figured it out yet that life doesn't calm down as we get older? Jobs, family, social obligations . . . they're never going to go away. If anything, they multiply! If you're waiting for a clear schedule, you're fooling yourself. The time is now, and in the case of *Prevention*'s Shortcuts workouts, it's often literally *right now*. Seriously, there is nothing so expensive, time-consuming, or overwhelming in this book that you need to "find the right time" to start. As you'll see in Chapter 3, you barely even need any equipment. All you need are dumbbells, which you might already own—and if you don't, there's a pair waiting for you at Target. Stop on your way home from work tomorrow and grab 'em.

"I can't get motivated." People feel most motivated when they feel rewarded. The awesome thing about the ultraquick *Prevention*'s Shortcuts workouts is that they provide instant gratification. In just 10 minutes, you'll be rewarded with instant energy, stress reduction, mood lift, and that special satisfaction that comes with checking something off your to-do list. And, as I explained in Chapter 1, even the big, long-term motivating rewards of exercise—like dropping a dress size, getting off blood pressure meds, and lowering cholesterol—will come to you faster than they would if you were doing longer, traditional workouts. Knowing this will help you keep moving toward your goals. Speaking of goals, setting good ones can get even the least-motivated exerciser in gear. Check out my goal-setting (and reward-giving) advice in Chapter 3.

"I blew it . . . again." When you miss your regular step class, it feels like a big deal because that was your one scheduled exercise time for the day. Miss it and 30-plus minutes of exercise time go out the window. If you miss one of your *Prevention*'s Shortcuts workouts, no great shakes. Just grab the other two later in the day. At the end of the day, you'll have missed only 10 minutes of workout time. As you'll discover as you go through the workouts in Parts 2 and 3, with *Prevention*'s Shortcuts, it's almost impossible to really "blow it" because you'll always be able to say you at least did *something*.

SHAPE YOUR LIFE TO GET IN SHAPE

People always say, "You're so lucky to be in such great shape." Well, luck has nothing to do with it! Not only do I map out my days to include exercise breaks, but I have also organized my life so I'm always ready to get up and take advantage of *Prevention*'s Shortcuts when the opportunity presents itself. I teach my clients to do the same.

For example, I teach women to "bundle their busywork" into one convenient time of day, like the lunch hour. By doing your bills and miscellaneous paperwork at your desk while you eat lunch, you free up 20 or 30 minutes at the end of the day for exercise. Other tricks:

- Take advantage of time-saving technology such as online banking, bill paying, and post office services.

- Buy two pairs of workout shoes, one for the office and one for home, so you're always good to go. I even keep a pair in my car, just in case I find time when I'm on the road.

- Piggyback *Prevention*'s Shortcuts workouts to your favorite never-miss activities, like watching *Grey's Anatomy* or your midafternoon latte break.

- Have a standing appointment with a workout buddy. If it's an always-there, can't-miss appointment, you'll just do it. Besides, you would never stand up a friend, but you would definitely stand up yourself.

- Rather than sit for hours (and hours) at kids' sports practices, do *Prevention*'s Shortcuts. I do cardio walking workouts from Chapter 4 during swim team practice in the summer. During my son's hockey practices in the winter, I can do any of this book's dumbbell workouts at the gym attached to the ice rink.

- Save yourself from the laundry. I do laundry on weekends. Period. Even with three kids. Everyone in the family should have five shirts and five pairs of pants they like for the week. If there's anything they *need*, they'd better throw it in the hamper for the weekend. This will save you hours.

Through such simple strategies, which I like to call Lifestyle Shortcuts, exercise becomes a part of the fabric of your life, instead of something requiring a complete overhaul of your life plan. This is the "magic bullet" women are always asking me for. Everyone wants to know "What is the least I can do?" or "What is good enough when my schedule is insane?" I tell them what I'm telling you in this book: You must adopt a "better than nothing" attitude! If every day you burn just 10 extra calories—the amount you can burn during 60 seconds of exercise (like doing one of the 1-Minute Wonder workouts found throughout this book), you will burn off 10 pounds in 10 years. Sounds like nothing, right? But realize that the average woman puts on about 10 pounds every decade of her adult life. She says, "Gee, I put on 10 pounds in my thirties and 10 pounds in my forties. Where are these pounds coming from?" I'll tell you where: from creeping inactivity and the idea that just a minute (or 10) of activity here and there isn't worth doing. Well, do the math: These 1-Minute Wonders can prevent you from gaining 10 pounds each decade of your adult life. How's that for being worth it? That's why you'll find lots more Lifestyle Shortcuts and 1-Minute Wonders scattered throughout the pages of this book.

So let's get started! The first step is a little self-analysis. What do you love to do? What do you hate? What obstacles seem to always trip you up en route to getting fit? What do you really want from an exercise program? By answering these few questions, you can pinpoint the *Prevention*'s Shortcuts workouts that will work best for you.

Take the following quizzes, checking off the answers that apply to you (it's okay to check more than one). Then read the analysis immediately following each segment for specific training advice and workouts to try.

QUIZ 1: WHAT WORKS FOR YOU?

Let's take a walk down memory lane. Like millions of Americans, you've likely started and dropped multiple exercise programs (even if they consisted of just a vow to walk every day). By identifying what has worked, you can increase your chances of making a program stick this time. How would you complete the following sentences? The answers will help you navigate the *Prevention's* Shortcuts workout system to find the routines best suited to what you love to do.

The exercise I stuck with the longest was . . .
   a. A walking program
   b. Strength training (at a gym or at home)
   c. A group exercise class
   d. Morning yoga

a. If you answered walking, that's no surprise. Most of us master it by age 2, and it's something we can hopefully do 'til we're 102. Plus it works! A landmark Harvard study of nearly 40,000 women over age 45 found that those who walked, even leisurely, for as little as 1 hour per week were *half* as likely to have a heart attack as those who rarely walked at all. If your walking shoes now spend more time parked in the closet than pounding the pavement, it's probably because you got a little bored or didn't see results. The *Prevention's* Shortcuts cardio walking workouts in Chapter 4 will fix both those problems.

b. Strength training is essential for maintaining shapely muscles and a highly charged metabolism, but it's easy to fall into a rut and stop seeing results. *Prevention's* Shortcuts solves that problem by offering a wide variety of moves (see Part 2) to mix and match. By surprising your muscles with new moves every 2 to 3 weeks, you stay firm and strong. I've also included specific programs geared toward women's most common problem spots in Part 3.

c. People who thrive in class situations tend to feed off the group energy and crave very specific exercise advice. You'll find nearly 50 specific workouts in this book, so there'll never be a question of what to do next. I'd also encourage you to find a friend (or two) to work out with, so you can keep it social. Instead of meeting your pals for double-chocolate mochas, make a date to do a quickie cardio workout like the ones in Chapter 4. Then reward yourselves with fat-free lattes afterward.

d. If yoga was your favorite thing, you probably loved the way it made you feel strong and flexible and serene all at the same time. You probably didn't love having to rearrange your day to make it to an hour-long class at a specific time of day. Check out the three quickie workouts in Chapter 12 that will let you keep what you love about yoga without what you don't.

I love exercise that makes me feel . . .
    a. Focused
    b. Serene
    c. Energized
    d. Pleasantly tired

a. There's nothing quite like "being in the moment" during an exercise routine, when your mind is blissfully clear of all distractions and you're homed in on how your body moves and feels. If that's the type of mind-body connection you crave, take a crack at the cardio interval workouts in Chapter 4 and the challenging combination moves in Chapter 6.

b. Some people love yoga for its well-documented stress-relieving powers, but as you've likely discovered, most women don't lose weight on Downward-Facing Dog alone. For the best results, try a routine that blends cardio, flexibility, and combination workouts (see page 150 for one of my favorites)—it will promote strength, grace, *and weight loss.*

c. *Prevention*'s Shortcuts workouts are well suited for women who love the energy boost a good exercise routine provides. The best part: Because each workout is just 10 minutes long, you can keep yourself buzzing throughout the day without ever worrying about burning out like you may with longer programs.

d. Like me, you probably love the good kind of tired a really tough workout provides, but you don't always have 50 minutes for a butt-kicking cardio class. That's why I included some 1-Minute Wonders and Chapter 4's high-energy interval workouts in the *Prevention*'s Shortcuts program. You'll fry fat, blow out stress, and finish feeling pleasantly spent. Check out the cardio workouts in Chapter 4 and the plateau busters in Chapter 6 to see what I mean.

As we age, balance and flexibility are the first things to go. *Prevention*'s Shortcuts can restore them. Check out the programs in Chapter 12. Because these routines are grounded in yoga fundamentals, you'll also infuse those supple muscles with strength and shape.

A nonexercise activity that I never miss is . . .
   a. My favorite prime-time television show
   b. Friday evening happy hour
   c. Church, synagogue, or other prayer service
   d. Saturday-morning yard sales
   e. Nightly reading (newspapers, magazines, novels)

a. I believe in linking exercise to the can't-miss activities in your life. If you love watching TV (nothing wrong with admitting guilty pleasures), why not work in *Prevention's* Shortcuts during a 30-minute show? For every half hour of show time, you can count on 7 to 10 minutes of advertisements. If you watch 2 hours of TV a night (and nearly everyone does), you can sneak in an entire workout without missing a minute.

b. I hear you! After a tough week, there's nothing like unwinding with friends for a few laughs. Go ahead and keep your occasional drink-and-chip gatherings. But also try a different way to blow off steam. Ask those friends to meet you at a local park for an end-of-day cardio walking workout. They might balk at first, but after a few jaunts in the fresh evening air, they may be hooked on a healthy new high.

c. There's a long tradition of walking meditation, as repetitive exercise helps clear the mind and allow spiritual focus. Your body is also a gift given to you from God. What better way to show appreciation for this precious gift and connect with your creator than to take care of yourself through exercise? If you're a spiritual person, choose exercises that allow you to be meditative and forge a deeper mind-body connection. I recommend the workouts in Chapters 4 and 12, which are built on a foundation of walking and yoga.

d. The best part of digging through a yard sale is discovering hidden treasures. Believe it or not, exercise can be just like that. Try this: Peruse Part 2 until you see a move that makes you go "hmmm." Do that move. Then page through and find another. Repeat for 10 minutes, three times a day.

e. Nothing like wind-down time at the end of the day. Here's an easy way to sneak in *Prevention*'s Shortcuts workouts. Grab your reading stack. Go upstairs. Do the moves in Chapter 12. Then settle in for your evening read. These gentle, repetitive moves will take your muscles through their full range of motion, so your body can relax comfortably while you read. You'll go to bed that night with the satisfaction of knowing you did something good for your body as well as your mind.

QUIZ 2: WHAT'S HOLDING YOU BACK?

Most women suffer from what I call the Type E personality. They try to be Everything to Everybody and end up lacking Energy. Sound familiar? If that's the case, you have to overcome your emotional barriers before you can take charge of your life. This quiz will help.

When I'm exercising, I feel . . .
    a. Guilty
    b. Happy
    c. Frazzled
    d. Frustrated
    e. Relieved

a. Here's the deal: You will never stick to an exercise program if it makes you feel guilty. If you feel like exercise is taking precious time away from your family, you'll never feel anything but bad about it. So it's time to reframe it. With all due respect to Einstein, here's my own personal energy equation: movement = stress relief = increased energy. Taking small amounts of time away from your family to exercise gives you *more* energy to enjoy being with them. With *Prevention*'s Shortcuts, you can also tell your family (and yourself), "It's just 10 minutes!" and every woman deserves that. Good-bye guilt.

b. Good for you! Take all the opportunities you can to do *Prevention*'s Shortcuts workouts and feel happy all day long.

c. If you feel just as harried on the treadmill as you do at the office, you need to change your exercise attitude. Rather than viewing your workout as another big job to do, think of it as a break for your brain. Remember, 10 minutes is all it takes, so you don't have to stress about all the work you've left undone on your desk or the dishes sitting in the sink. Plan three 10-minute respites, or Shortcut Slots, throughout the day—ideally, one midmorning, one midafternoon, and one in the evening. These brain breaks will leave you feeling refreshed instead of frazzled.

d. When women feel frustrated from exercise, it's usually due to two reasons: They're struggling with the exercise itself, so they feel incompetent; or they don't see results, so they don't see the point. The two are often related and come from trying to do too much too soon. The antidote is success. Start with just one *Prevention's* Shortcuts workout a day. When you've made that happen for 7 days straight, add another, then another. Nothing is more motivating (and satisfying) than the realization that you can do it.

e. You love to exercise; you just don't make it happen as often as you'd like. Follow the advice for answers c and d to make more time for the movement you crave.

When I start exercising, my family . . .

    a. Joins in
    b. Supports me 100 percent—they even help with the household chores
    c. Gives me positive lip service but doesn't offer much assistance
    d. Seems to resent the time I take away from them
    e. Rolls their eyes and says, "Not again . . ."

a & b. Who could ask for more? My kids and husband love to work out, so I encourage them every chance I get. Recruit the whole family—for whatever they're up for! If they're supportive but inactive themselves, invite them to join you for one or two *Prevention's* Shortcuts workouts a week. Before long, you may have company every time you exercise.

c. It's hard to feel like your family is really supportive when they don't lift a finger to help you, I know. But let's give them the benefit of the doubt. Do you tell them *specifically* how to help you? I honestly believe that husbands and kids have biological blind spots to dog hair on the furniture, dirty dishes on the counters, and laundry on the floor. Tell your family exactly what you need. Say "I'm going to work out for 10 minutes, so do me a favor and chop these vegetables for dinner." Don't expect them to read your mind.

d & e. Change can be scary for families. Kids and husbands often see you in a very specific way. When you start messing with that image by starting an exercise program, they get nervous and may even try to sabotage your efforts. Ease their minds by not making a huge production out of what you're doing. Say "I'm doing this for me, to feel better and have more energy. It's only going to take 10 minutes here and there, so don't sweat it." If you don't make a big deal out of it, they won't either. More important, your exercise is a shining example to your kids and grandkids. Remember, kids are influenced less by what you say and more by what you do. They tend to adopt their parents' way of life. And you're setting a very healthy example.

Among the people closest to me, the following exercise regularly:
a. My husband
b. My kids/grandkids
c. My co-workers
d. My friends
e. Nobody close to me exercises regularly

a & b. The family that plays together stays together. If your family is involved in sports and activities at certain times, try to sneak in your *Prevention's* Shortcuts workouts around those same times. Even better, join in each other's activities when you can.

c. Most Americans spend at least a third of their day at the office, so active co-workers can be a big blessing. Tag along for their noontime walking workouts. Or when the weather is bad, bring in your favorite *Prevention's* Shortcuts workouts and commandeer an empty conference room for an impromptu gym.

d. Exercise is the perfect excuse for hanging out with friends. Activity loves company!

e. Sometimes when I'm coaching clients about making healthy lifestyle changes, they look at me incredulously and exclaim, "What you're saying is that I need all new friends!" Well, I won't tell you to dump your family or friends because they're not active. But no woman is an island. If you are completely surrounded by people who are inactive, it will be that much harder for you to keep moving. My advice: Look around and find just one active friend. It may be a co-worker you don't know well who walks at lunchtime. Maybe it's a neighbor. Strike up a conversation and ask to join her occasionally. Having one person in your life who really understands your efforts can make all the difference.

QUIZ 3: WHAT *NEVER* WORKS?

We all have exercises we just don't like to do. Me? I hate running outside in the bitter-cold Minnesota winters. Don't get me wrong, I love nature. But when it's less than 25°F out, I'm staying indoors, no matter how good the fresh air and sunshine may be for me. It's a big fat waste of my time to try to psych myself up for something I just don't enjoy. I'm not going to do it. Here's your chance to be honest and figure out what it is you just won't do (and, of course, what you will).

I can never . . .
    a. Drag myself out of bed on cold, dark mornings
    b. Motivate myself to work out at the end of a long workday
    c. Squeeze a workout into my lunch hour
    d. Get to an exercise class regularly, no matter when it is
    e. Exercise by myself, anytime

a. I really don't believe anybody is born desiring to get up at 5:00 a.m. and go do a workout. But for millions of busy women, the morning is the only time of day they have to themselves, so I encourage all women to squeeze in a little a.m. activity. If you're not a morning person, forget getting up at the crack of dawn for an hour on the elliptical trainer. Instead, set your clock just 10 minutes earlier than you usually get up and do a quickie workout like the one on page 85. You'll still be well rested, and you'll have the satisfaction of knowing you have a workout under your belt before you've even started the day.

b. My cowriter Selene Yeager relates, "All I want to do is go home and eat!" But sometimes, after 5:00 p.m. is her only free time. Her solution: "I have my husband start dinner, and I commit myself to a superefficient, superfast workout like the combination moves in Chapter 6. My muscles get a great workout, and I don't end up eating any later than if I'd skipped exercising entirely."

c. If your boss frowns on long lunches, it can be virtually impossible to squeeze a 30- or 45-minute workout into your lunch hour. So stop trying. Do a 10-minute *Prevention's* Shortcuts workout instead. That'll leave you plenty of time to grab a bite to eat and bring it back to your desk without worrying about running late.

d. Obviously, getting to a class won't be a problem with the *Prevention's* Shortcuts program. But be honest with yourself: Can you make it to haircut and pedicure appointments on time without fail? Most people who miss exercise class do so because they aren't making it a priority. The *Prevention's* Shortcuts workouts are 10 minutes. There's no reason you should miss them, no matter what comes up. Write them in your schedule, and make a commitment to get them done.

e. Lots of people hate exercising by themselves because the time seems to drag. *Prevention's* Shortcuts workouts are so short that that shouldn't be an issue. But if it is, ask your husband or kids to join you. If no one's available, put on your favorite tunes. Music is a surefire way to make time fly. As a bonus, you get to break out all that great techno (or punk rock or country) that nobody seems to love as much as you!

I hate . . .
   a. Running
   b. Lifting weights
   c. Group cardio classes
   d. Yoga
   e. Sports

a, b & d. Everyone has some type of exercise they just don't like, generally because it's either too hard, too boring, or a combination of the two. Among my clients, running tops the list, though plenty of women complain about resistance training, too. But what if you just had to do those things for a few minutes? Many of my clients hate running and strength training because they get bored after 10 minutes. It's excruciating for them to look down this giant list of exercises and feel like they're going to be there all day. It's amazing how they perk up when they realize they can get the same results with less. I challenge you to give the workouts you usually hate a try using *Prevention's* Shortcuts. You may have a change of heart.

c & e. Group sports and classes make you feel miserable? Don't do them! There are plenty of ways to get fit that have nothing to do with keeping a beat or hitting a ball. About 50 of them are right here. Now, don't you feel better?

The worst part about working out is . . .
    a. The sweat
    b. The clothes
    c. The perky people
    d. Feeling clumsy or awkward
    e. The aches and pains

a. I'll be honest. If you sweat easily, there may be no way around getting a little bit of a glisten during even a 10-minute *Prevention's* Shortcuts workout. But, as you'll see once you start doing the *Prevention's* Shortcuts routines, you don't have to be sopping through sweat towels to get in shape. You also can minimize your sweat exposure by wearing moisture-wicking clothes made with light synthetic fabrics like Coolmax. See Chapter 3 for more gear advice.

b. We've come a lo-o-ong way from thongs and leotards! From Nike to Athleta, there are so many wonderful companies making stylish, comfortable workout wear for ladies of all shapes and sizes. Chapter 3 will help you find clothes you'll love. You'll want to wear them everywhere!

c, d & e. More often than not, I find these complaints rolled together in the same breath. No doubt, when you're feeling miserable, there's nothing worse than being surrounded by perky, smiling faces. There is no reason to feel miserable when you're working out, no matter how out of shape you are. Americans are stuck on the mind-set that more is better and "no pain, no gain." What I love about the *Prevention's* Shortcuts approach is that it forces people who hate working out to do what they absolutely need to do: Start slowly! Turn to Chapter 5, and do just one of the workouts in that section. I promise you, it won't beat you up or make you feel bad about yourself. Do the same thing tomorrow. Once you've done three or four without feeling bad, add another. Slow and steady always wins.

QUIZ 4: BUSY VERSUS ACTIVE

Are you really so busy it is impossible to squeeze in exercise, or do low-priority items eat up hours of your average day? If the president of the United States has 10 minutes to spare, so do you! Let's take a look at your life and find the places you may be killing precious time.

I spend ___ minutes in the car every day (including to and from work, errands, etc.).
   a. < 30
   b. 30 to 40
   c. 40 to 50
   d. 50 to 60
   e. 60+

a & b. Give yourself a pat on the back. You've figured out how to live in our car-o-holic society without being buried in your bucket seat half the day. If you spend less than 40 minutes in your car every day, chances are it's not eating into your exercise time. The only exception: if that 40 minutes is an amalgamation of small trips running here and there. I try to "bundle" my errands to minimize car time. When possible, park in a common spot (like between the dry cleaners and the grocery store) and walk to your destinations. This is one of the Lifestyle Shortcuts that can help enhance the *Prevention*'s Shortcuts program.

c & d. Between 40 and 60 minutes is inching into the danger zone. Pick 3 days (including 1 weekend day), and in one column write down every trip you make and how long it takes. In another column, prioritize the trips from A to C, with A being essential, B important, and C being borderline. Eliminate at least one C trip from each day. My favorite tips: Sign up for online banking (saves hours every month!); buy stamps online; take advantage of dry-cleaning services that pick up and drop off garments at your office. With a little planning, you can eliminate wasted gas, energy, and time in the car.

e. Spending an hour or two in the car every day can take a giant bite out of your fitness time. If you simply can't change your commute, take the advice above to eliminate any unnecessary car time. Also investigate your options. Can you do flextime once or twice a week to avoid the rush-hour traffic and cut your commute? Can you telecommute occasionally? What if you started carpooling (it's amazing how much paperwork you can get done when someone else drives!)? You don't know until you ask.

During the average day, I wait 10 or more minutes for . . .
   a. My kids to get ready for school
   b. Client appointments
   c. Callbacks or responses to e-mails
   d. Dinner (other meals) to be ready
   e. Service (on hold on the phone, waiting in line at the store, etc.)

a. I'll say it again: Morning is prime exercise time for busy women. Stop screeching at the kids to get moving. If you're standing around waiting for them, it means you're the one with time to kill. Provided you're all getting out the door on time, let them know you'll be doing your morning workout and that they'd better be ready by the time you're ready to roll. Set an egg timer for them if you need to. But don't waste another moment of precious time standing around drumming your fingers.

b. Obviously, you can't hurry clients along. But you can always be prepared to take action when plans go awry. I keep a pair of sneakers in my car, so when a client unexpectedly cancels or is running way behind, I can do a *Prevention's* Shortcuts cardio walking workout to blow off steam instead of sitting and stewing. Returning calls, filling out paperwork, even a few moments of stretching or meditating are other great go-to tasks when you find yourself with unexpected time on your hands.

c. Studies show employees waste countless hours every day with e-mail. Try this: Designate three or four specific times in the day as "e-mail times." Then use those 15- or 20-minute periods to send out e-mail queries and reply to ones that have come in for you. Aim for first thing in the morning, 11:30 a.m., 2:30 p.m., and 4:30 p.m. Your important work will get accomplished, and you won't find yourself killing time waiting for responses.

d. Most of my clients feel ridiculous doing lunges in the kitchen while waiting for the chicken to bake. So instead of trying to turn dinnertime into an hour of power, use this time to relax, catch up with the family, read the paper, pay bills, and so forth, so you have more free time to do a *Prevention*'s Shortcuts workout after dinner once you've rested and digested.

e. Three words: Internet, Internet, Internet. Just as modern conveniences have stolen activity from our lives and helped make us fat, they can give us time back to help make us trim. Use the Web wisely to eliminate busywork from your day, and use that time for exercise instead.

Okay, I'll admit it. I spend too much time . . .
   a. Watching TV
   b. Surfing the Web
   c. Poring over junk mail
   d. Chatting on the phone
   e. Eating, drinking, food-related socializing

a. When I meet clients who watch more than 2 hours of TV a day, I ask them why they're so interested in living everyone's lives but their own. Life on TV, even so-called reality TV, isn't real. At least, it's not your life. Nice for a brief escape, but if you spend too much time there, you are letting your own life pass you by! There's no sugarcoating this one: Too much TV makes you fat. And the average American spends an astonishing 4 hours a day watching TV! In a 6-year study of more than 50,000 women, Harvard researchers found that for every 2 hours spent watching television, women were 23 percent more likely to be obese. Break the cycle by planning your TV time. Pick two shows a night, and turn off the TV when they're done. Even better, buy a TiVo (the new toy in my home). You can record what you like, watch it at your convenience, and zap through the commercials to save almost 20 minutes every hour.

b. Like TV, the Internet can be a dangerous time sucker if used mindlessly. You sit down "just to check e-mail," and suddenly it's 2 hours later. Some of my clients surf the Web while they watch TV to kill two guilty pleasures in an hour (an idea I love). Or you can keep your dumbbells by your computer and work out while you surf. Surf for 10 minutes. Do a *Prevention*'s Shortcuts workout. Surf. Work out. And so on.

c. This is *definitely* one you can do while watching TV. Put all your mail in an easy-to-carry basket, then take the whole thing to the TV room so you can sift through it during your favorite shows. Bonus: It'll keep your hands busy, so you'll be less likely to snack at the same time.

d. Call your friends during daily mindless tasks such as loading and unloading the dishwasher, poring over mail (see above), and filing papers. Even better, meet in person once or twice a week to catch up during a cardio walking workout around the neighborhood.

e. Eating has replaced active hobbies like bowling and gardening in America—and it shows! It's time to put food back into its proper place as something we enjoy during family time and when we're hungry, not something we seek out simply because we're bored. To help you take control of your eating habits, see the Clean-Eating Shortcuts in Chapter 3. The first step to reducing mindless eating is being aware of it. The second is filling that time with something more worthwhile. I recommend the exercise routines in Part 3.

QUIZ 5: WHAT ARE YOUR GOALS?

Ask yourself: "Why am I really reading this book?" Are you tired of seeing an image in the mirror that doesn't reflect who you really feel you are? Have you outgrown all your jeans? Does playing with your kids or grandkids leave you winded? Knowing your goals helps you define exactly what you need to do to achieve them. They can also serve as motivation for getting started and sticking with the program.

I want to get fit because . . .
- a. I want to be able to keep up with my kids/grandkids.
- b. I want to look better in my favorite clothes.
- c. I'm unhappy with all the weight I've put on.
- d. I want to lower my blood pressure/cholesterol/blood sugar.
- e. I need to look better for a wedding/reunion/other big event.

a & d. Many of my clients want to get fit for practical reasons. They need energy to keep up with their kids, or they're worried that their high cholesterol or blood pressure might keep them from being around for their grandkids. Exercise can help you toward your fitness goals and has nothing but good side effects (see "Just What the Doctor Ordered . . . " on page 34). The *Prevention's* Shortcuts workouts that will work best for you are the ones designed to encourage weight loss, such as those in Chapter 5, and those that keep your body strong and limber, like those in Chapters 12 and 13.

b. Sounds like you have a few pounds inching on here and there, or sometime—seemingly overnight—your body proportions changed. It happens! Over time, we naturally lose lean muscle tissue and replace it with fat. Plus, as our hormone levels change, our excess weight starts shifting from our hips to our bellies. That doesn't mean you have to be a passive bystander as your weight creeps up and your muscle tone heads south! Try the total body-shaping workouts in Chapter 6, as well as the spot toners in Part 3, to hit your specific problem areas.

c. It didn't come on overnight, so it won't magically disappear in a week. But by using the workouts in Chapter 5, you can start peeling off those added pounds and drop up to two dress sizes in 8 weeks.

e. See the advice for answer c. If your 20th reunion is 4 weeks away, you can drop a dress size or two and look and feel better, but you're not going to lose 30 pounds without doing something extreme and unhealthy—and even that probably won't work. Use this event as a springboard for a new you. It is the real pounds and inches lost, real habits forming, and real lifestyle changes that make you the person you want to be.

When I look in the mirror, I want to see . . .
    a. My old self
    b. Confidence
    c. Muscle tone
    d. My cheekbones
    e. Sparkle

a. First you have to answer, what's changed? Was your old self thinner? Happier? More energetic? Adopting the *Prevention's* Shortcuts program will turn back time on muscle loss and weight gain, so you'll feel thinner, stronger, and more energetic.

JUST WHAT THE DOCTOR ORDERED . . .

If all the health benefits of exercise were available in a pill, the pharmacies would be sold out in a day. By being active every day for less time than it takes to watch a rerun of *Friends*, you can:

- **Lose weight.** Even mellow exercise burns three times the number of calories used by sitting on the sofa working the remote. You must burn 3,500 calories to lose a pound. That's 500 calories a day to lose a pound per week (or 250 calories burned if you eat 250 fewer calories, which is easy to do if you use the Clean-Eating Shortcuts in Chapter 3). At the end of the day, the amount of weight you lose depends on the number of calories you burn. Keeping it simple makes it feel more doable. Remember, weight loss is calories in versus calories out. It's simple math!

- **Bring down blood pressure.** Physical activity is inversely related to the progressive buildup of plaque in your carotid arteries (the all-important ones that deliver blood to your brain). Studies show that even people who just golf or garden on the weekends have clearer arteries than those who do nothing.

- **Beat diabetes.** Duke University researchers found that regular exercise improves blood sugar metabolism by almost 25 percent. A single bout of exercise improves blood sugar metabolism immediately.

- **Lower cholesterol.** It's no secret that losing

As I always tell clients, "I don't necessarily want to be younger. I just want to feel younger." Chronological age is different than your body age! *Prevention*'s Shortcuts will help you make the latter younger.

b. See the answer to a. Success breeds confidence, and *Prevention*'s Shortcuts is designed to make it easier than ever for you to succeed at getting strong and losing those stubborn pounds. After you finish this evaluation, turn to Chapter 3 to schedule your workouts and get started today.

c. Open the book to Part 3 and get started! So long as you aren't carrying more than 5 to 10 extra pounds, you'll turn those flabby spots into fabulous spots in just 3 or 4 weeks.

weight helps cut bad cholesterol levels. But exercise by itself, with or without weight loss, is still effective. A study from Duke revealed that exercise changes the structure of the protein particles that carry cholesterol, making it harder for them to damage the arteries and set the stage for heart disease.

- **Feel happier.** A growing body of research confirms the blues-beating power of exercise. Research shows exercise works as well as anti-depressant drugs for improving well-being. A single walk around the neighborhood can boost the mood of someone who's even clinically depressed.

- **Stop smoking.** Yep, even otherwise health-minded people still smoke cigarettes some-times, not because they're lazy or bad people, but because they're addicted. Moving your behind helps you kick those butts without gaining lots of excess weight, according to Brown University research.

- **Bank more beats.** The average inactive person's heart beats 70 to 75 times per minute—more than a beat per second. A fit, active person's heart is so strong that it can squeeze out about 25 percent more blood with every beat, so it only needs to pump about 50 times per minute. That adds up to 36,000 fewer beats every single day—or 13 million fewer beats each year.

d. Whether you put extra padding in the cheeks you sit on or the cheeks surrounding your smile is a matter of genetics. But the good news is that the fat you store in your face is often the first to go when you lose weight. By doing *Prevention*'s Shortcuts workouts and cleaning up your diet (see Chapter 3), you can make those cheekbones shine through.

e. Women are like lightbulbs. Without energy, there's no illumination. Our hair is lifeless, our skin drab; there are little dark circles under our eyes—you get the picture! Why have you lost your sparkle? Are you really low on energy and down? Or are you deprived of energizers like sleep, good food, or physical movement? I'm guessing the latter. The *Prevention*'s Shortcuts system will help you reenergize by putting movement back into your life all throughout the day and by helping you make smart food choices. The result: You'll feel better, sleep better, and see a glowing, vibrant woman staring back at you next time you look in the mirror.

The one item of clothing I can't wait to wear is . . .
   a. Jeans
   b. Sleeveless top
   c. Shorts/skirt
   d. A belt
   e. Tankini

a–e. Belly, butt, thighs, arms. We all have areas we camouflage with clothes. No more! Everyone knows you can't "spot reduce" (i.e., take an inch off your thighs solely by doing 1,000 leg lifts). But you *can* spot tone and firm up those flabby muscles to make problem areas look better. When you combine spot toning with fat loss, any body part can be shaped up to put on display! Check out the programs in Part 3 to address your specific goals.

1-MINUTE WONDER
LET YOUR FEET DO THE WALKING

Next time you have a complex message to send to a colleague, skip the six or seven e-mail exchanges and just walk over and discuss the issue face-to-face. Stanford University researchers calculated that if you were to walk across the building and back to your office to talk to someone instead of spending the same 2 minutes sending an e-mail, you could save 11 pounds over 10 years.

CHAPTER 3

Map Out
Your Shortcuts

Basketball living legend Shaquille O'Neal once said, "Excellence is not a singular act, but a habit. You are what you repeatedly do." By picking up this book and getting this far, you have already committed a series of excellent acts. With this chapter, I'm going to help you turn those acts into habits by weaving exercise, good eating, and positive thinking into the fabric of your life. I'll show you what to buy, how to set goals, and how to measure your progress and stay on track. I'll also provide some tips about healthy eating to help speed you on the way to your destination. Let's start with what you need. Though you could do all these exercises at the gym, I've designed the *Prevention*'s Shortcuts workouts to be done in the comfort of your home or even in your cubicle at work. Every move can be done with the bare minimum of equipment. Hit your local sporting goods store and get started today.

EQUIPMENT SHORT LIST

Dumbbells. Hand weights are essential equipment for the *Prevention*'s Shortcuts system. Because you'll be working muscle groups of all strengths and sizes, from your thighs to your triceps, I strongly recommend you buy three pairs of dumbbells: a light pair (3 to 5 pounds), a medium pair (8 to 10 pounds), and a heavy pair (12 to 15 pounds). You can find weights in these ranges in the sporting goods department of most major retail stores. To shape up stubborn body parts, you need to use a weight that is heavy enough to fatigue your muscles. Studies show the majority of people choose weights that are too light to do the job. So don't shy away from a pair of weights because they feel a little heavy and you're afraid of building big muscles. Women don't get "muscle bound" without spending many hours in the weight room and, often, taking supplements. But without sufficiently heavy weights, you won't get the lean, jiggle-free muscle tone you crave.

Keep your weights in a convenient place where you can't miss them, such as by your dresser or in front of your full-length mirror, as a constant reminder to pick them up and get moving.

Shoes. Your feet support every inch of your body, so quality shoes are a must. Doing even brisk 10-minute walks in shabby, unsupportive tennis sneaks can cause foot pain, shin pain, knee pain, and connective tissue problems like Achilles tendinitis and plantar fasciitis (heel pain). What's more, you'll walk faster, feel springier, and perform better in a quality pair of shoes. I recommend buying a good pair of running shoes, because even if you're not a runner, the *Prevention's* Shortcuts program prescribes lots of cardio walking workouts, including some short bursts of speed equal to very fast walking or basic jogging. Running shoes will provide the right amount of strength, cushioning, and stability to protect your feet.

Though you can buy dumbbells from any store that carries them, I recommend buying your running shoes from a specialty sports-shoe store. The staff there is trained to measure your feet, examine how you stand and move in shoes, and find a pair that fits your specific biomechanical needs. Many shops will even let you take them for a "test run" on an in-store treadmill or even around the block before you buy. Though good running shoes aren't cheap (usually around $70), it's a great idea to buy two pairs: one pair to keep at work and one for home. It's a small investment for the convenience of always being ready to exercise without having to schlep your shoes back and forth to and from work every day.

Clothes. Remember when women's workout attire consisted of either a leotard and thong bodysuit or black tights and a giant baggy shirt? We've come a long way, baby! Today's workout clothes from women's activewear companies like Athleta, Nike, adidas, lululemon athletica, New Balance, and lucy are so flattering and fashionable, many of my clients wear them not just to exercise but also for running errands, shopping, and even to work. My cowriter, Selene Yeager, confesses to being an "Athleta addict." "I'm a busy working mom, so I need to be able to work out and then run off to a meeting without having to change all my clothes. I live in Athleta tank tops, shirts, capris, and shoes. And everywhere I go, people compliment my clothes. I love seeing the startled looks on their faces when I tell them they're 'workout clothes.' I think it's a downer to throw on some ratty shirt and shorts to go work out. Clothes that feel great and look good make you feel good about yourself."

I'll second that! If the activewear selection at your favorite department store leaves you cold, check out the goods from places like Athleta.com, Activasports.com, or lucy.com. If you buy nothing else, at least invest in some comfortable, supportive bra tops so everything stays put when you pump up the pace around the neighborhood.

Optional accessories. You need nothing more than hand weights and shoes to do the *Prevention*'s Shortcuts workouts. But there are a few niceties that can make your home workouts even nicer. One is a sticky yoga mat. This slim, "grippy" exercise mat provides a stable, nonslip surface for you to perform your yoga, strength training, and stretching. It also can be easily rolled up and stored. You can find one in most sporting goods stores and large department stores.

The other accessory I love (and live by) is a heart rate monitor—a device that works like an electrocardiograph, measuring how many times your heart beats per minute. To lose weight and get in shape, you need to raise your heart rate into aerobic, fat-burning territory (see Chapter 4 for more details on how heart rate monitors work and how you can use them with the *Prevention*'s Shortcuts system). Though there are other methods—such as rating your breathing or using the "rate of perceived exertion"—to measure how hard your heart is pumping, a heart rate monitor is a no-brainer way to gauge the work your body is doing so you can meet your fitness and weight loss goals fast.

My clients are usually hooked on heart rate training after the first try. For them, it's like having me along on every walk. One client, Katie, who lost 15 pounds and more than two dress sizes, explains it like this: "I always thought I was walking at the right pace, but once I started watching my heart rate, I learned that I often wasn't working hard enough to burn all the calories I wanted to burn. My monitor reminds me to push myself a little more and keeps me moving toward my goals."

Heart rate monitors are great for any exercise from walking to swimming. You can get a basic model for about $80 at Polarusa.com.

Cleanup. During the hot summer months, you may perspire a little even during short workouts. For a quick, "no sweat" cleanup, keep a box of baby wipes and extra antiperspirant at work. You can wipe your face, feet, and underarms and feel fresh and clean in less than a minute.

SET GREAT GOALS

Every exerciser needs goals. They keep you motivated and clarify what you are trying to achieve with your efforts. As you attain each goal, you gain encouragement and further motivation. Here is how to set your goals and achieve the goals you set.

Make them measurable. A vague goal such as "I want to be fit" gives you nothing to shoot for. "I want to lose 2 inches off my waist by August 1," on the other hand, is a meaningful, measurable goal. If you're still struggling with goal setting, go back and review your responses to the quizzes in Chapter 2. Then explore them more deeply. Suppose you checked "I'm unhappy with all the weight I've put on" as the main reason you want to get fit. Visualize why that weight is making you unhappy. Is it because you have a closet full of clothes you can't wear? Is it because you can't play with your kids or grandkids without feeling pooped? Then set a concrete goal: "I want to be able to play with the kids in the park for an hour straight by May 30" or "I want to wear my favorite jeans by September." Being able to close that zipper is a pretty measurable goal!

Whatever goals you set, give yourself a reasonable time frame to accomplish them. Everyone wants to drop 15 pounds by Friday, but it simply isn't realistic. The maximum healthy, sustainable weight loss is 2 pounds a week. Those first 2 pounds won't elicit cries of "Wow, how much weight have you lost?" But after 8 weeks, you'll have dropped two sizes, and those results will be obvious to everyone. And unlike those quick-fix diets, where people wind up noticing how you put all your weight right back on, this will be a permanent improvement.

Set "stepping stone" goals. If your goal is a biggie—say, more than a 25-pound weight loss—set short-term weekly or monthly goals to keep you moving in the right direction without getting discouraged. Aiming for 1 to 2 pounds a week is a healthy, reasonable, and, more important, sustainable goal. Weekly goals will also help you adjust your plan if you're not seeing progress. For instance, if you decide to lose a pound a week and you step on the scale two Sundays in a row without the needle budging, you know you need to take a closer look at your eating and your adherence to the *Prevention*'s Shortcuts program.

Create a plan. A concrete action plan is imperative for making your goals a reality. I like to start by writing reasonable, achievable "I will" statements—for example, "I will set my alarm 10 minutes earlier than usual 4 days this week to ensure I fit in my morning exercise" or "I will add two fruits to my diet every day." Setting simple, reasonable goals will help you stay upbeat and on track. Putting it down on paper helps you to be more objective and concrete about your goals. It also helps you to better analyze your progress as you move forward. The *Prevention*'s Shortcuts workout logs in Part 3 are perfect plan-setting tools. In fact, I've done most of the work for you. Just fill them out to stay on track.

Reward your successes. I'm a big believer in self-nurturing, and there's no better time to nurture yourself than when you're shedding some of your old, comfortable lifestyle habits to make room for a new, healthier way of life. Even positive change can be stressful, so be kind to yourself by acknowledging your progress. I generally try to stay away from food rewards. There's nothing wrong with the occasional bowl of ice cream; what I don't like is the emphasis it places on satisfaction through food and food alone. Instead, buy yourself a brow wax, some new lipstick or lip gloss, or some cute workout shoes, or treat yourself to a hot stone massage.

Practice patience . . . and forgiveness. There will be days when everything goes to the dogs—days when you have raging PMS, get swamped at work, and eat two slices of cold pizza before you take off your coat and cook dinner. Nobody's perfect. Even the most dedicated exercisers have setbacks; the difference between those who succeed long-term and those who don't is how they deal with them. If you immediately think "I've blown it, I'm so fat, why bother?" that overwhelming sense of failure will make it harder to get yourself back on track. Successful exercisers shrug off the workout that never was and the occasional overeating and go back to making healthy choices right away. Stay positive and keep moving forward. As author and speaker Zig Ziglar would say: It's not what happens to you that determines how far you will go in life, it is how you handle what happens to you.

Finally, remember that it's not enough just to set these goals. You need to put them in action! "I'll do it later" turns into never. So as you're writing your goals, add *when* you're going to put them in action. Be specific. *Action* is one word that guarantees results!

FINDING THE GAPS

Now that everything's in place, it's time to fit *Prevention*'s Shortcuts into your day. For most of these programs, you're going to need three or four 10-minute windows, or Shortcut Slots, in your day. Ideally, schedule one in the morning, one in the afternoon, and one in the evening to keep your calorie-burning metabolism revved all day long. Let's look at "a day in the life" of some typical women to find some natural activity breaks.

Check out the following *Prevention*'s Shortcuts Lifestyle Makeovers. Here I help two women find (and fill) the gaps in their lives. When you're done reviewing their makeovers, try your own. Write out a typical day using the formats shown here. Using the examples below, highlight the spots where *Prevention*'s Shortcuts workouts fit perfectly. Then schedule them into your calendar and make them happen!

The Working Mom

Susie is a 41-year-old mother of three boys (all under the age of 5) who also holds down a full-time sales job. Though she's doing a pretty good job of sticking to a healthy diet, she still has a little spare tire around her middle that she'd love to lose. She would also like to tone up from head to toe, but she hates the idea of going to a gym and feels too tired at the end of the day to force herself to work out. She also doesn't want her workout time to take away from her family time: "I want to be there for them whenever possible."

TYPICAL WEEKDAY (SCHEDULE ON OPPOSITE PAGE)

Shortcut Slot #1: 7:00 a.m. Many working women already set the alarm for the crack of dawn, so a long morning workout is out of the question. But most of us can arise just 10 or 20 minutes earlier without feeling any ill effects. Try waking at 6:45 a.m. and squeezing in one of the cardio walking workouts from Chapter 4 to jump-start your day.

Clean-Eating Shortcut: 6:30 p.m. Skip the extra bites while you clean up after dinner; they can add up to hundreds of calories a day. To keep from eating scraps, try chewing bubble gum while you clean up the dishes.

Shortcut Slot #2: 7:00 p.m. When you're at home, get the family to try some *Prevention*'s Shortcuts exercises with you. Pick a belly-flattening workout from

Typical Weekday

Shortcut
SLOT #1

7 AM
7:00 Wake, shower, feed kids, and help them as much as I have time for.
7:30 Au pair takes over; I leave for work.
8:00 Arrive at work.

8 AM
8:00–11:30 Sales calls in and out of the office; desk work.

9 AM

10 AM

11 AM
11:30 Lunch. I eat most often in the office, but I love to go out to lunch—it's relaxing.

12 PM
12:30 Sales calls in and out of office.

1 PM

2 PM

3 PM

4 PM

5 PM
5:30–6:00 Arrive back home.

6 PM
6:00 Weight Watchers meetings on Mondays. Otherwise, help au pair with dinner and usually make my own dinner now since watching weight.

6:30–7:00 Dishes and cleanup. Sometimes "pick" at meal or steal another bite of dinner.

Shortcut
CLEAN EATING

7 PM
7:00 Play with boys, watch TV, or do home computer work. Try to squeeze in time for myself, if possible: maybe go running, maybe go out for happy hour, maybe play golf.

Shortcut
SLOT #2

8 PM

9 PM
9:00 Put boys to bed.

9:30 Finally have time alone to clean up or relax.

Shortcut
SLOT #3

10 PM
10:00 In bed; watch TV.

10:30 Lights out.

Chapter 8. Get on the floor and let the boys have fun, too! Save happy hour for once a month only. Try squeezing in another 10-minute cardio workout—you can take it outdoors if it's nice outside. Add a workout from Chapter 10. These are fun moves that the boys may try to mimic. If your husband or au pair will watch the boys, string together three *Prevention's* Shortcuts workouts—cardio, booty, and flat tummy or a plateau buster from Chapter 6.

Shortcut Slot #3: 9:30 p.m. Wind down with one of the flexibility workouts from Chapter 12. Use these yoga poses to relax and feel centered before bed.

PREVENTION'S SHORTCUTS CONCLUSION: Great day! If all goes well, you've squeezed in as many as five workouts! Guaranteed total-body toning.

TYPICAL WEEKEND (SCHEDULE ON OPPOSITE PAGE)

Shortcut Slot #1: 7:00 to 8:00 a.m. We all love to catch up on sleep on the weekends. But lying in bed too long can throw us out of sync and leave us more tired instead of refreshed. Try waking up just 10 minutes earlier, and squeeze in a *Prevention's* Shortcuts belly-flattening workout from Chapter 8. You'll still get your extra z's, but you'll start the day with your motor running.

Shortcut Slot #2: 9:00 a.m. to noon. Too often parents end up just standing on the sidelines while they make sure their kids get exercise and playtime. Make at least 10 minutes of these 3 hours cardio time for you. Try one of the cardio walking workouts to kick it into high gear. If you can spare another 10 minutes, try a workout from Chapter 6, which includes multijoint moves to target all muscle groups in 10 minutes.

Shortcut Slot #3: 1:00 to 3:00 p.m. Another great opportunity to squeeze in 10 minutes between lunch and chores. Try a Beautiful Booty workout from Chapter 10 to work the legs and get the heart rate up!

PREVENTION'S SHORTCUTS CONCLUSION: Relax—you deserve it. You've already squeezed in 30 to 40 minutes of focused exercise today!

Add It Up!

Using *Prevention's* Shortcuts, Susie, 41, lost a total of 30 pounds—12 of them in the first 6 weeks on the program—and dropped from a size 14 to a size 6! "This is the

Typical Weekend

Saturday

7 AM	7:00–8:00 Wake up—unless the kids wake me up sooner.	**3 PM**	3:00 Playtime with the boys.
8 AM	8:00–9:00 Kids watch TV; make breakfast for everyone.	**4 PM**	
9 AM	9:00 Sometimes try to go on an activity with boys, go to a park, friend's house, swimming lessons, or sometimes hang out at home.	**5 PM**	
10 AM		**6 PM**	6:00 Dinner.
11 AM		**7 PM**	
12 PM	Noon. Come home for lunch or eat out.	**8 PM**	
1 PM	1:00–3:00 Nap time and quiet time; I run around and get stuff done.	**9 PM**	9:00 Bedtime for boys but usually takes until at least 9:30 to go to bed. Many times, we get together with friends and take the boys. Try to get home by 9:30.
2 PM		**10 PM**	10:00–11:00 Bedtime for us.

Shortcut SLOT #1

Shortcut SLOT #2

Shortcut SLOT #3

first time I actually had fun exercising. I had never enjoyed exercising because I previously thought it was too hard and it made me tired. Now I actually look forward to doing my workouts because I have finally had success with the weight loss and want to keep it off."

The Stay-at-Home Mom

Meghan, 32, whom you met in Chapter 1, is a married stay-at-home mom with four kids, including a 2-year-old daughter and three teenage

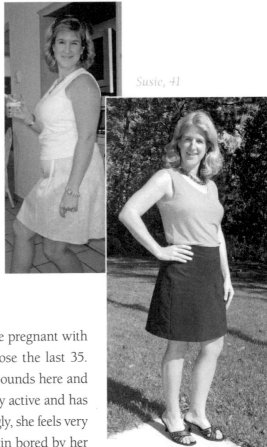

Susie, 41

stepsons. She gained 60 pounds while pregnant with her daughter and has struggled to lose the last 35. During the past 2 years, she lost 10 pounds here and there but struggled to stay consistently active and has put the weight back on. Not surprisingly, she feels very overwhelmed and sometimes just plain bored by her daily demands of laundry, errands, housecleaning, and work. Though she tries to eat healthfully, her diet often falls apart in the evening, when she's tired and hungry. "I start snacking around 5:00 or 6:00. Then I decide I need a glass of wine, which turns into two or three, and before you know it, I'm snacking on what's most convenient, like pizza, chips, or something microwaveable."

TYPICAL WEEKDAY 1: ONLY ONE KID HOME—BOYS AT GRANDMOM'S HOUSE (SCHEDULE ON OPPOSITE PAGE)

Shortcut Slot #1: 7:00 a.m. Exercise can set the tone for a demanding day, increasing your energy level and instilling in you a sense of accomplishment. Start with a cardio walking workout from Chapter 4. Get on the treadmill for 10 minutes with a bottle of water—turn on *Today* and breathe! Chores can wait until you finish your

Typical Weekday 1

only one kid home—boys at Grandmom's house

Shortcut SLOT #1

7 AM

7:00 Wake up, do morning chores (dog, dishes, laundry, etc.) while watching the news.

Lifestyle Shortcut

7:30 Have cup of coffee and read the paper.

8 AM

8:00 Shower.

8:30 Get daughter up.

Shortcut SLOT #2

9 AM

9:00 Feed her breakfast; empty dishwasher.

9:30–10:30 Get paperwork done, make phone calls in family room while daughter plays next to me.

10 AM

10:30–11:30 Go to mom-and-child gym class.

11 AM

12 PM

Noon. Feed daughter lunch.

12:30 Get her ready for nap.

Shortcut SLOT #3

1 PM

1:00–3:30 Eat my lunch, finish chores around house, finish phone calls, schedule appointments, return e-mails, work on charity stuff.

2 PM

3 PM

3:30 Get daughter up.

4 PM

4:00–5:30 Go to park to play.

Shortcut SLOT #4

5 PM

6 PM

6:00 Feed daughter dinner and hang out in kitchen while she eats, organizing my piles or reading a magazine or the mail.

7 PM

7:00 Read books with daughter; give her a bath.

7:30 Start bedtime routine.

8 PM

8:00 Put daughter to bed.

8:00–10:00 Eat my dinner, watch TV with husband, finish any leftover laundry and dishes, talk on the phone.

Shortcut SLOT #5

9 PM

10 PM

10:00 Watch news and go to bed.

Prevention's Shortcuts workout. Try Strong and Steady (page 86) on Mondays and Wednesdays, Need for Speed (page 85) on Tuesday, Fast and Focused (page 86) on Thursday, and Pyramid Power (page 87) on Friday.

Lifestyle Shortcut: 7:30 a.m. Try shifting your respite with coffee and the paper until 7:45 or until your daughter is eating breakfast.

Shortcut Slot #2: 9:00 a.m. You don't have to sit and wait for your daughter to be done eating breakfast. If she's a slow eater, do one of the Chapter 8 ab workouts (rotate between workouts A, B, and C) while she's eating. Or have a little playtime on the floor when she's done eating, and squeeze in your ab exercises then.

Shortcut Slot #3: 1:00 to 3:30 p.m. Take a *Prevention's* Shortcut as soon as your daughter is down for her nap, before you get distracted. Try a different workout from Chapter 4 or one from Chapter 5 to get your heart pumping with weights.

Shortcut Slot #4: 4:00 to 5:30 p.m. While your daughter plays, you play. Do another of the cardio walking workouts from Chapter 4. For extra credit, you can also push her on a swing or in her stroller. If it's raining and you stay home, do a 10-minute strength and Cardio Quick Take workout from Chapter 10. Or try a few 1-Minute Wonders. If you need to get out of the house, go to the mall and do your walking workout there.

Shortcut Slot #5: 8:00 to 10:00 p.m. Evening TV time is the *best* time to stretch. You're warmed up from the activity of the day. You're usually tired, so you want a low-energy activity. And often you're in a room with a nice carpeted floor, conducive to stretching your body out. Do one of the Chapter 12 flexibility workouts, or, if you do feel more energetic, pick a quick total-body workout from Chapter 5. Invite your husband to join you. It's only 10 minutes, and you are watching TV for 2 hours. You could get it done in the first few commercials!

PREVENTION'S SHORTCUTS CONCLUSION: You just got in at least 40 minutes, and maybe even 50 minutes, of exercise in an otherwise crammed day!

TYPICAL WEEKDAY 2: BOYS AT GRANDMOM'S HOUSE, DAUGHTER GOES TO A.M. PRESCHOOL (SCHEDULE ON OPPOSITE PAGE)

Shortcut Slot #1: 7:00 a.m. Same recommendation as yesterday; work out while you watch the news.

Typical Weekday 2

boys at Grandmom's house; daughter goes to a.m. preschool

Shortcut SLOT #1

7
AM

7:00 Wake up, do morning chores (dog, dishes, laundry, etc.) while watching the news.

7:30 Have cup of coffee and read the paper.

3
PM

3:30 Get daughter up.

8
AM

8:00 Get daughter up.

8:30 Feed her breakfast; empty dishwasher.

4
PM

4:00–5:30 Go to park to play.

Shortcut SLOT #4

Shortcut SLOT #2

9
AM

9:00 Take daughter to preschool.

9:30–noon Run errands and do anything else I need to do without my daughter.

5
PM

10
AM

6
PM

6:00 Feed daughter dinner and hang out in kitchen while she eats, organizing my piles or reading a magazine or the mail.

11
AM

7
PM

7:00 Read books with daughter; give her a bath.

7:30 Start bedtime routine.

12
PM

Noon. Pick up daughter and feed her lunch.

12:30 Get her ready for nap.

8
PM

8:00 Put daughter to bed.

8:00–10:00 Eat my dinner, watch TV with husband, finish laundry or dishes, talk on the phone.

Shortcut SLOT #5

Shortcut SLOT #3

1
PM

1:00–3:30 Eat my lunch, finish chores around house, finish phone calls, schedule appointments, return e-mails, work on charity stuff.

9
PM

2
PM

10
PM

10:00 Watch news and go to bed.

Lifestyle Shortcut: 7:30 a.m. Same as yesterday.

Shortcut Slot #2: 9:30 a.m. to noon. For women with families, solo time is like gold, so I understand that you don't have the luxury to spend it all on an hour-long workout. But you can definitely squeeze in a *Prevention's* Shortcut in a 2½-hour block of free time. I'd recommend one of the Chapter 10 Beautiful Booty workouts to use your large muscle groups and get your heart pumping. There are days when you have to juggle the demands of four kids—10 minutes of focused strength training is an easy task compared to that!

Shortcut Slot #3: 1:00 to 3:30 p.m. Just like yesterday, start a *Prevention's* Shortcut as soon as your daughter is down for her nap, before you get distracted. Try a different workout from Chapter 4 or 5 to get your heart pumping with weights.

Shortcut Slot #4: 4:00 to 5:30 p.m. Same as yesterday. Don't just sit there while your daughter plays. Join in!

Shortcut Slot #5: 8:00 to 10:00 p.m. Same as yesterday. TV time can be active time.

PREVENTION'S SHORTCUTS CONCLUSION: Another day when you did a lot *more* than the recommended minimum 30 minutes of exercise. Great job!

TYPICAL WEEKEND: ALL FOUR KIDS AT HOME (SCHEDULE ON OPPOSITE PAGE)

Shortcut Slot #1: 7:00 a.m. Your dog can be your greatest weight-loss ally! Don't just open the door and let the dog walk around the yard. Take this opportunity to do a 10-minute cardio walk—better yet, do two if you aren't in a hurry to be somewhere. This is a golden opportunity to get your blood pumping!

Shortcut Slot #2: 1:30 to 3:00 p.m. Squeeze 10 or 20 minutes in here during your free time—best if you commit to doing one or two *Prevention's* Shortcuts right after you put your daughter down for a nap, before you get pulled in other directions. Do 10 minutes of abs from Chapter 8 and 10 minutes of strength training from Chapter 5 for a real energy boost. Let the family know your expectation that they give you a little time to yourself. Not a lot to ask!

PREVENTION'S SHORTCUTS CONCLUSION: Enjoy your family time on weekend evenings. Feel good that you already snuck in 20 to 40 minutes of high-quality exercise today!

Typical Weekend

all four kids at home

7 AM	7:00 Wake up, take dog out.	**3** PM	3:00 Get daughter up from nap.
8 AM	8:00 Have coffee and read the paper. 8:30–9:30 Get daughter up and make breakfast for whomever is up.	**4** PM	
9 AM	9:30–noon Run errands, do housework, play with daughter, family activities with other kids when awake.	**5** PM	
10 AM		**6** PM	6:30 Feed daughter.
11 AM		**7** PM	7:00 Get daughter ready for bed/bath. 7:30 Start bedtime ritual.
12 PM	Noon. Feed family lunch.	**8** PM	8:00 Put daughter to bed. 8:00–11:00 Eat dinner, watch movies with older kids, husband, etc.
1 PM	1:00 Put daughter down for nap. 1:30-3:00 Do me-time things (shop, read, etc.) or drive older kids to and from sports and friends.	**9** PM	
2 PM		**10** PM	10:00 Watch news and go to bed.

Shortcut SLOT #1

Shortcut SLOT #2

Add It Up!

Meghan has dropped 25 pounds and is just 10 pounds away from her prepregnancy weight. By the end of a month, she'd lost 10 pounds; and in less than 2 months, she'd lost 15. The best part: "I have more energy than ever before, and I'm not taking any time away from my family."

You can see how easy it is for even the most time-strapped woman to find 30, 40, and even 50 minutes to take care of herself every day. But it doesn't happen by accident! Though you can (and should) be spontaneously active, you can't always count on "seizing the moment" when it arises. You must *plan your workouts* just as you would any important appointment or meeting. Put it into your day planner. Write it on the calendar. Make it an official, nonnegotiable part of your day. If you can, try to be consistent in when you exercise, as well. If you always exercise on the same days at the same time, your routine will become a fixture in your life, not a whim. Inserting exercise into your busy schedule will be an adjustment at first, but with consistency, *not* exercising will begin to feel as unnatural as not brushing your teeth or reading the mail.

Finally, when you start planning out your day, be a little selfish! Women are notorious for putting everyone's needs and desires before their own. As a result, they end up with built-up resentment that leaves them short-tempered with the very people they claim to be sacrificing for to make happy! (I do it, too.) That's why I believe you need to fill your own needs and desires first, so you're in better shape to fill others' needs and desires. Women tell me all the time, "My family won't let me exercise." Don't make it an option. Find the times that work for you, and they will adjust.

Here's a trick that works like magic for my family. I hang an erasable whiteboard (the kind they use in offices and many classrooms now) in our mudroom, where it's immediately visible when you come in the door. On it, I write the schedule for the week. It includes all my meetings and my husband's as well, our kids' sports practices, after-school activities, and so on. Each day, I write when I'm going to do my workouts. It's on the board, everyone knows it, and not once has anyone ever whined about it or questioned it. Try it for yourself. It works. And trust me, you'll be better for it. Running around on empty, feeling overspent and underappreciated, isn't good for you or your family. They'll be happier when you're happy, too.

PREVENTION'S SHORTCUTS PLANNING

There's one thing the big weight loss chains have in common: diaries. Experts know that you're much more likely to succeed if you make yourself accountable by putting your actions in writing. I realize you don't have time to write down every exercise you do, so I've done the work for you by creating workout logs to keep you on track and help you follow your progress. Just copy those pages, which you'll find in each workout chapter in Parts 2 and 3, and check off the workouts you perform. There's even space for you to record your goals and make other important notes, such as your starting weight, your current weight, the place where you performed your workout (in the family room on the treadmill, at the soccer field, etc.), how you felt about your workout—anything you think will help keep you motivated. These logs will ensure that you're following the program as recommended and will serve as a reminder that you're on the path to a new, healthy, strong you. By keeping you consistent, they'll also speed your results. Consistent exercise improves not only your overall health and fitness but also your appearance, energy level, and social life. You'll reap countless psychological benefits as well, such as confidence, self-esteem, and relief from depression, anxiety, and stress. Now that's worth noting!

CLEAN-EATING SHORTCUTS

Weight loss is a simple fuel-efficiency equation: How much you put in your tank – How much you burn = How much you lose. With the *Prevention's* Shortcuts system, you'll be revving your engine several times a day, boosting your metabolism to help burn more fuel from the time you roll out of bed until you hit the sheets. To help you reach your weight-loss goals even faster, you have to address the other side of the equation: food.

This analogy demonstrates exactly how you should approach food: as fuel. Just as Americans are trying to keep the planet healthy by replacing dirty fossil fuels with cleaner-burning alternatives, it's time to make your body healthier by removing the additives, preservatives, processed sugars, carbs, and general junk from your diet. Stay calm. I'm not saying you can never buy Ben & Jerry's or Frosted Flakes again. I still buy doughnuts, chips, and ice cream. But here's the key: These are not staples. These are treats. My family and I enjoy them occasionally. The rest of the time, we fuel ourselves by following what I call Clean-Eating Shortcuts. Follow these diet shortcuts 80 percent of the time, allowing yourself to bend the rules on special occasions the other 20 percent, and you'll be golden!

Don't Diet

If diets worked, everybody would be slim. Seriously! Look around you. Did all those superstrict low-fat diets from the early 1990s work? Did the low-carb craze of the past 5 or 6 years work? Are all those people ordering 11-ounce steaks and gnawing on beef jerky suddenly slimmer? No! At best, diets work temporarily by eliminating entire macronutrients like fat or carbohydrates. But they never, ever work long-term. What's more, there is something fundamentally wrong when Americans are chowing down on bacon and cheesesteaks but are afraid to eat apples and carrots because they're "high in carbs"! There is something fundamentally wrong with Americans spending billions of dollars on low-carb products packaged in bags and boxes with lots of additives, fake sugar alcohols, and ingredients even Rhodes scholars can't pronounce, while completely skipping past the fresh fruit and whole grain aisles at the grocery store. Yet that's *exactly* what popular diets have you do.

Enough! Here's all you need to know. Losing weight is about portion control, not the exclusion of food groups. I'll make it easy for you. Divide your plate into four sections. Fill one-quarter with a healthy protein food like fish, poultry, or lean red meat; fill one-quarter with a whole grain like brown rice; and fill the other two quarters with vegetables and fruit. Add a glass of milk, and you're set. Still hungry? Serve yourself additional helpings of veggies until you're satisfied. Vegetables are naturally low in calories and high in fiber, which helps you feel full.

You can also use this "handy" portion scale to size up your servings at restaurants, at home, or wherever you eat.

Fist = 1 cup of rice or pasta; 1 piece of fruit

Thumb = 1 ounce of cheese

Tip of thumb (to bottom of nail) = 1 teaspoon of butter

Palm = 1 serving of meat, poultry, fish

Cupped handful = 1 serving of cereal, chips, pretzels

Generally speaking, one serving of each food group should suffice for one woman (remember that veggies are unlimited). The first few times you rightsize your servings, it's not going to look like much food on your plate. But portion distortion is the underlying reason for much of our weight gain, so we need to retrain our eyes to recognize the amounts our bodies really need. If you like the look of a full dish, simply put your food on a smaller plate to make you feel like you're getting more. But I promise, once you start eating right-size servings, you'll

be surprised at how little food it takes to feel satisfied. To avoid overeating when you're at a restaurant, simply rightsize your meal, then immediately ask for a to-go container, so you can finish the rest at another meal.

This, and the other *Prevention's* Shortcuts eating advice, is not some temporary quick fix or crash diet. It's a lifestyle change that will deliver lasting results.

Eat from Plants, Trees, and Animals

When you look at your plate, you should see food that looks like it came from a living thing: a plant, animal, or tree (not from a box, bag, or drive-thru). That's fruits, veggies, meats, poultry, fish, and dairy. The more recognizable it is—like broccoli, carrots, chicken breasts, mangoes, and fish—the better! As food becomes more processed and less immediately identifiable, you should eat it less often. For example, bread, pasta, and cereal are okay, but choose whole grains that resemble the food that grows on a farm, like oatmeal and brown rice, over those like Froot Loops that are unrecognizable as anything from nature. Completely processed foods such as cakes and candies should be eaten very sparingly.

For some women, following this advice means tweaking their grocery lists and resisting the occasional urge to visit the vending machine with a fistful of quarters. For others, it's a complete sea change from the way they're used to shopping and eating. Here are some tips to smooth the transition, no matter where you start.

Shop the perimeter first. Grocery stores stock the most vibrant, healthy foods around the perimeter, so shop there first. Fill your cart with a colorful array of fresh and frozen fruits and vegetables; lean meats, poultry, and fish; dairy foods; and whole grains. By the time you reach the inside aisles, where the packaged and processed foods are, your cart should be pretty full. Top it off with healthy packaged foods like oatmeal, nuts, whole grain cereal, tortillas (without trans fats), tuna, pasta, and spices.

Go beyond bananas. Fruit is one of the healthiest, most satisfying foods. Unfortunately, many people never make it past orange juice and bananas. Those are great, of course—I freeze sliced banana "coins" for a treat—but the more variety, the better. Here are some of my favorite tips for getting more fruit in your diet.

- Puree canned apricots, peaches, or pears (not in heavy syrup) and serve warm over whole grain waffles.
- Add dried fruits to cereal or homemade muffins.
- Add fruit to a green salad. My favorites are pears, apples, and red grapes.
- Make fruit kebabs for the family. Use melon, pineapple, berries, and—yes— bananas. Roll in coconut sprinkles for added flavor.
- Dip strawberries in a small amount of chocolate or whipped cream for a special treat.
- Mash strawberries with a little Splenda and eat with light vanilla ice cream.
- Make fruit smoothies. Use a little yogurt, fresh or frozen fruit, and soy milk or orange juice. Delicious!

Buy it ready to eat. All that healthy food will do you no good if it rots in your fridge while you eat a bag of White Castle burgers because they were faster and you were in a hurry. For fast, fresh food, check out the prewashed, prebagged fruits and veggies like salads and fresh chopped fruit salads. Check the deli section for presliced, marinated cutlets. Buy freshly sliced turkey breast for sandwiches. I'm not shunning convenience, just the excess fat, cholesterol, sodium, and calories that come with traditional fast food.

Wake Up Your Metabolism

If you do nothing else for your brain and body, eat breakfast! Study after study has shown that even the simplest morning meal—a bowl of whole grain cereal, some skim milk, a handful of strawberries—lengthens attention span, sharpens fact recall, and elevates mood. Though most of the research is done on kids, the same holds true for adults. Cognitive skills like focus and recall are greatly improved when you start your day with proper fuel.

Breakfast eaters are also slimmer than a.m. fasters. Research over the past 30 years has shown without fail that breakfast is a key component of weight control. In fact, breakfast skippers are 4½ times more likely to be obese than folks who regularly eat a good morning meal, according to a recently published study in the *American Journal of Epidemiology*. Why? Because your body slows down while you sleep, and it doesn't speed back up again until you put fuel in it. That's why exercising in the morning on an empty stomach (a "weight loss" trick I've seen so many clients try) never works. After about 7 hours of sleep, about 70 percent of your body's glycogen stores are depleted. That means by morning, you have less than a third of your usual stored carbs to fuel your muscles. "Great!" you think. "Then my exercise will burn more fat!" Sounds logical. But it's not true. As any nutritionist will tell you, fat burns in a carbohydrate flame. You need carbs to help break down and burn your stored fats. Otherwise, your capacity to burn body fat slows down. Eating even a small snack can reignite your fat-burning metabolism.

While many women skimp on breakfast because they're "not hungry" or "too busy," if you want to lose weight, you need to make your morning meal a priority. Ideally, it should be at least the same size as dinner, if not bigger (and dinner, of course, should be smaller). By eating 25 to 30 percent of your day's calories in the morning, you'll start the day well fueled and be less likely to snack all afternoon or, worse, binge at night. Some of my favorite Shortcut breakfasts for at home or on-the-go are

- Whole grain cereal—cold or hot—like oatmeal with skim milk and dried fruit and nuts
- Toasted whole grain bread with natural peanut butter and jelly
- Fruit or protein smoothie
- Yogurt—add crushed nuts for extra crunch!
- Whole grain frozen waffles with fruit
- Trail mix in a zipper-lock bag (mix up cold cereal, nuts, dried fruit, pretzels, etc.)
- Breakfast burrito (put cheese and some refried beans on a tortilla, heat in the microwave, add some salsa, and roll it up)
- String cheese and a piece of fruit
- A quick egg white omelet—add leftover veggies or meat
- Peanut butter and sliced banana on whole grain toast

One word of caution: Avoid starting the day on a sugar binge. (I've always thought the word *muffin* was invented so we wouldn't feel guilty about eating cake for breakfast!) Sugary cereals, breakfast bars, muffins, and pastries may give you a temporary boost, but they won't fill you up long enough to sustain you through the morning. A healthy breakfast will.

Snack Smart

We are a snack food nation. According to a national survey on Americans' food habits, 60 percent of us eat snack food regularly, and we eat 20 percent of our calories from snacks—that's one-fifth of our daily food intake. If we're going to subsist on snacks, we must make smarter choices. Chips, candy, and snack cakes have to go. It boils down to a little discipline and preparation. When it comes to food, failing to plan is planning to fail. Stock your pantry, and don't let convenience overtake health. If you don't see it, you won't eat it! Don't buy foods that you don't want to eat. If you have an uncontrollable craving for chips or ice cream on a Friday night, you can always go to the store to get a small bag or carton to split with the family while you watch a movie. That way, your indulgence becomes a conscious decision instead of mindless munching.

ADD FLAX

Healthy fats are the cornerstone of any successful weight loss eating plan, and they don't get much healthier than flax. Flax (either the seeds or the oil pressed from the seeds) is rich in good-for-you omega-3 fatty acids, dietary fiber, protein, and antioxidants called lignans. And it tastes good! Flax's pleasant, nutty flavor complements soups, salads, cereals, pasta dishes, and almost any baked good.

Studies show that flaxseed may be one of the best foods for controlling cholesterol. It helps keep the heart healthy, controls blood sugar, and may even fight cancer. Eating more of the healthy fats in flax will help you eat less, lose weight, and prevent disease.

I recommend adding it to your foods in either oil or ground-up seed form. Add a tablespoon or two to oatmeal, smoothies, and pancakes. Bake it into muffins. Drizzle it on salads. Stir it into yogurt. You'll find whole flaxseed in almost all grocery stores, as well as many health food stores and natural foods markets. You can store it at room temperature for up to a year. Just grind the seeds in a coffee grinder as you use them. You can also buy it already ground if you use it within a few days. That's what I do to save time.

Follow the same rules in your workplace: If your co-worker insists on keeping a candy jar handy, kindly ask her to push it out of sight. A recent study from the University of Illinois found that office workers who had candy on their desks ate about three more pieces every day than those who stashed it in their desk drawers, and they ate 5½ more pieces than workers who put it all the way across the room on a shelf. By moving the dish out of arm's reach, you'll both eat less!

We have to take a stand on feeding ourselves and our families. Smart snacking doesn't have to be tedious. It can be fun, fast, and delicious. Here are a few on-the-go goodies I know you'll enjoy.

- Trail mix. Combine nuts, pretzels, whole grain cereals, a few M&M'S (they add a nice chocolatey treat to the mix; just don't go overboard), and dried fruit like raisins in a large plastic storage container. Fill snack bags as you need them. This simple snack is a great source of vitamins, minerals, carbohydrates, healthy fats, and protein.

- Crunchy granola bars. The chewy kinds often contain unhealthy fats and are not as nutritious.

- Baked snack foods. Baked chips, crackers, or pretzels are fine for an occasional snack. Just be sure they have no trans fats.

- Carrots and hummus or low-fat ranch dressing.

- A zipper-lock bag of peanut butter and some apple slices for dipping.

- Seasonal fruit. Keep a big bowl in the kitchen where it's easy to grab and go. Apples and bananas are available year-round. Also try peaches, pears, grapes, and clementines.

- Homemade peanut butter sandwich cookies. Take 2 graham crackers and spread them with peanut butter. Put them together like a sandwich.

- Cinnamon toast (made from whole grain bread) with fruit.

- Ants on a log. Celery sticks filled with light cream cheese or peanut butter and lined with raisins.

- Hard-cooked eggs, lightly sprinkled with salt or seasoning.

- A small bowl of whole grain cereal with fat-free milk.

- Nuked sweet potatoes. Thinly slice a sweet potato, spread it out on a plate, sprinkle with salt and ground black pepper, and microwave for about 4 minutes. These "potato chips" are more filling than the fried bagged kind, and they're brimming with beta-carotene.

K.I.S.S.: Keep It Simple and Speedy

If you're convinced that takeout is the only way to save time, try this experiment: Next time you're cruising through the local drive-thru, time yourself from the moment you pull off the road to the moment you roll back onto the road. I guarantee

SUPER SNACKS

Each of these goodies will cure even the worst case of the munchies—for just 200 calories.

- 8 ounces fat-free yogurt with 1 tablespoon slivered almonds, ground flaxseed, or wheat germ

- 2 tablespoons raw or dry-roasted nuts or seeds of choice (sunflower or pumpkin seeds, slivered almonds, walnuts, pecans) with 2 tablespoons raisins or dried cranberries or cherries

- 1 cup raw veggie of choice dipped in 2 tablespoons reduced-fat ranch or blue cheese salad dressing

- 1 cup raw veggie of choice dipped in 1/2 cup hummus

- 1 medium apple with 1 thumb-size slice of cheese or 1 tablespoon peanut butter

- 2 hard-cooked eggs sprinkled with Parmesan cheese

- 1 packet plain oatmeal with 8 ounces fat-free milk

- 1 Nature Valley Granola Bar (super easy for carrying in briefcases, backpacks, or handbags)

- 1 Luna bar; my favorite flavor—iced oatmeal raisin

- 2 caramel-flavored rice cakes topped with 1 teaspoon hazelnut chocolate spread

- 3 cups air-popped popcorn sprinkled with 1 tablespoon garlic salt, seasoning salt, or freshly grated Parmesan cheese; use your kitchen mister and mist a wee bit of olive oil on them to hold the seasoning

- 1 slice whole wheat toast with 2 slices avocado, tomato, onion, sea salt, and pepper

you that the time you spend waiting in line, choosing your food, waiting for it to be slapped together and bagged, digging out money, counting your change, and checking your order will add up to 10 minutes—the time it would take to prepare a simple, healthy meal in your own kitchen. That's why I believe in cooking—and in cooking simply. I cook chicken breasts, add some fresh fruit and steamed vegetables, maybe a baked potato or brown rice, and there's dinner. Meals can be very basic and quick.

Here are 10 healthy *Prevention* magazine recipes that are ideal for the Shortcuts program. For each of them, the prep time is 10 minutes or less. Once you've assembled the ingredients, each dish either can be cooked in under 10 minutes or will be on the stove or in the oven or slow cooker long enough for you to fit in a 10-minute *Prevention*'s Shortcuts workout and get back to the kitchen before the meal is done. Shop on weekends to pick up all the ingredients you'll need. That way, you can easily throw together breakfast and lunch before you head to work and make dinner in no time after you return.

MIXED BERRY MUESLI

PREP TIME: 7 minutes

    8 ounces fat-free vanilla yogurt

    2 tablespoons quick-cooking oats

    2 tablespoons chopped walnuts

    ¼ cup blueberries

    ¼ cup raspberries

    ½ small cantaloupe, seeds removed

In a medium bowl, combine the yogurt and oats, mixing well. Fold in the walnuts, then gently fold in the blueberries and raspberries. Scoop into the melon and serve.

Makes 1 serving

PER SERVING: *451 calories, 18 g protein, 76 g carbohydrates, 11 g fat, 5 g saturated fat, 4 mg cholesterol, 7 g fiber, 192 mg sodium*

GREEN TEA, BLUEBERRY, AND BANANA SMOOTHIE

PREP TIME: 5 minutes

3 tablespoons water

1 green tea bag

2 teaspoons honey

1½ cups frozen blueberries

½ medium banana

¾ cup calcium-fortified light vanilla soy milk

In a small glass measuring cup or bowl, microwave the water on high until steaming hot. Add the tea bag and allow it to brew for 3 minutes, then remove. Stir the honey into the tea until it dissolves.

In a blender with ice-crushing ability, combine the berries, banana, and milk. Add the tea and blend on ice crush or highest setting until smooth. (Some blenders may require additional water to process the mixture.)

Pour smoothie into a tall glass and serve.

Makes 1 serving

PER SERVING: *299 calories, 5 g protein, 69 g carbohydrates, 3 g fat, 0 g saturated fat, 0 mg cholesterol, 8 g fiber, 74 mg sodium*

LEAN REUBEN

PREP TIME: 2 minutes
COOKING TIME: 7 minutes

> 2 slices seeded rye bread, toasted
>
> 2 tablespoons reduced-fat Thousand Island dressing
>
> 2 ounces Canadian bacon (2 slices)
>
> 1 cup fresh, canned, or jarred sauerkraut, drained
>
> 2 slices Swiss cheese

Preheat the oven to 400°F.

Spread each slice of bread with the dressing, and top with the bacon, sauerkraut, and cheese, in that order.

Place on a baking sheet and bake for 5 to 7 minutes. Serve open-faced.

Makes 2 sandwiches

PER SANDWICH: *280 calories, 17 g protein, 23 g carbohydrates, 13 g fat, 5 g saturated fat, 44 mg cholesterol, 3 g fiber, 1,032 mg sodium*

TRICOLOR PIZZA

PREP TIME: 5 minutes
COOKING TIME: 10 minutes

1 head broccoli, separated into small florets

2 prebaked regular or whole wheat pizza shells (12" diameter), such as Boboli

1 cup reduced-fat shredded mozzarella cheese

1 pint cherry tomatoes, halved

6 tablespoons grated Parmesan cheese

1 cup torn basil leaves (optional)

Preheat the oven to 500°F.

In a large pot of rapidly boiling water, cook the broccoli, uncovered, for 2 minutes, or until crisp-tender. Drain and set aside.

Place each pizza shell on a baking sheet. Sprinkle with the mozzarella, add an even layer of the tomatoes, and dot with the reserved broccoli.

Bake for 8 minutes, or until the crusts are golden brown and crisp. Remove and sprinkle with the Parmesan. Scatter the basil leaves on top, if desired. Cut each pizza into 6 slices and serve.

Makes 6 servings (2 slices each)

PER SERVING: 425 calories, 23 g protein, 53 g carbohydrates, 14 g fat, 6 g saturated fat, 26 mg cholesterol, 4 g fiber, 820 mg sodium

SPRING ORZO SALAD

PREP TIME: 10 minutes
COOKING TIME: 9 minutes

⅔ cup orzo

⅓ cup finely chopped red bell pepper

⅓ cup finely chopped orange bell pepper

⅓ cup finely chopped and seeded tomatoes

¼ cup quartered dry-packed sun-dried tomatoes

¼ cup chopped scallions

¼ cup chopped watercress

1 teaspoon minced garlic

2 teaspoons extra-virgin olive oil

⅓ cup crumbled reduced-fat feta cheese

2 teaspoons fresh lemon juice

Prepare the orzo according to package directions.

Meanwhile, in a medium bowl, mix the bell peppers, tomatoes, scallions, watercress, garlic, oil, cheese, and lemon juice.

Mix the orzo with the vegetable mixture until well combined. Season to taste with salt and ground black pepper. Serve immediately or refrigerate in a plastic container.

Makes 2 servings

PER SERVING: *343 calories, 14 g protein, 53 g carbohydrates, 9 g fat, 3 g saturated fat, 7 mg cholesterol, 4 g fiber, 461 mg sodium*

CHICKEN WITH CITRUS-AVOCADO SALSA

PREP TIME: 4 minutes
COOKING TIME: 15 minutes

4 boneless, skinless chicken breast halves

½ teaspoon + ⅛ teaspoon salt

1 ruby red grapefruit

1 avocado, peeled, pitted, and diced

4 radishes, thinly sliced

¼ cup chopped basil leaves + additional for garnish

Lettuce leaves (optional)

Place the chicken in a large saucepan with 4 cups water and ½ teaspoon salt. Bring to a boil over high heat. Turn off the heat and let the chicken sit, covered, for 15 minutes, or until a thermometer inserted in the thickest portion registers 160°F and the juices run clear.

Meanwhile, remove the peel and pith from the grapefruit with a knife. Working over a bowl to catch the juice, free each segment from the membrane and cut into bite-size pieces. Gently toss the grapefruit with its juice, the avocado, radishes, basil, and remaining ⅛ teaspoon salt.

Drain the chicken, discarding the liquid. Slice crosswise into ½" slices. Divide the citrus-avocado salsa into 4 portions and add a quarter of the chicken to each, drizzling the chicken with the salsa juice. If desired, serve over lettuce leaves and garnish with additional basil leaves.

Makes 4 servings

PER SERVING: *237 calories, 26 g protein, 9 g carbohydrates, 11 g fat, 2 g saturated fat, 66 mg cholesterol, 3 g fiber, 428 mg sodium*

ITALIAN HUNTER-STYLE CHICKEN

PREP TIME: 8 minutes
COOKING TIME: 7–9 hours

1 jar (26 ounces) marinara sauce

8 ounces shiitake mushrooms, stemmed and sliced ½" thick

2 large carrots, peeled and halved lengthwise, sliced ¼" thick (1 cup)

⅓ cup dry white wine

1 tablespoon chopped fresh thyme leaves or ½ teaspoon dried

¼ teaspoon fennel seed

¼ teaspoon crushed red pepper

4 skinless chicken drumsticks and thighs

2 small yellow squash, sliced into ¾"-thick rounds

Thin strips basil leaves (optional)

Thyme sprigs (optional)

In a 4-quart or larger slow cooker, combine the sauce, mushrooms, carrots, wine, thyme, fennel, and pepper. Add the chicken and toss to coat. Place the squash on top.

Cover and cook on low for 7 to 9 hours, or until the chicken and vegetables are tender. Serve with the sauce, and garnish with basil and thyme, if desired.

Makes 4 servings

PER SERVING: 330 calories, 31 g protein, 29 g carbohydrates, 9 g fat, 2 g saturated fat, 105 mg cholesterol, 6 g fiber, 900 mg sodium

STEAK BURGERS

PREP TIME: 10 minutes
COOKING TIME: 8 minutes

> 1½ pounds 96% lean ground beef
>
> 6 whole grain hamburger buns, sliced
>
> 6½ ounces reduced-fat Swiss cheese, sliced
>
> 6 leaves red or green leaf lettuce
>
> 6 tomato slices, ¼" thick
>
> 6 red onion slices, ⅛" thick
>
> 6 tablespoons chopped parsley
>
> ¼ cup steak sauce

Preheat an indoor or outdoor grill to the highest heat setting.

Shape the beef into 6 patties slightly larger in diameter than the buns (try not to overhandle or the meat will toughen). Season both sides of the patties with salt and freshly ground black pepper. Grill the patties for 2 to 4 minutes per side, or until they reach the desired doneness.

Meanwhile, place the buns on the grill and toast for 1 minute. Add 1 slice of the cheese to each patty to melt just before the burgers are done.

Assemble the burgers by placing a lettuce leaf on the bottom half of each bun, followed by a tomato slice, the burger, and an onion slice. Sprinkle with the parsley. Add 2 teaspoons of sauce to each burger. Top with the remaining buns.

Makes 6

PER SERVING: *321 calories, 35 g protein, 27 g carbohydrates, 10 g fat, 9 g saturated fat, 70 mg cholesterol, 4 g fiber, 441 mg sodium*

CRANBERRY-APRICOT PORK ROAST

PREP TIME: 10 minutes
COOKING TIME: 7–9 hours

1 can (16 ounces) whole-berry cranberry sauce

½ cup quartered dried apricots

½ teaspoon grated orange peel

¼ cup orange juice

1 large shallot, chopped (⅓ cup)

2 teaspoons cider vinegar

1 teaspoon mustard powder

1 teaspoon salt

1 teaspoon grated fresh ginger

2 pounds boneless pork loin roast, well trimmed

Snipped chives (optional)

In a 4-quart or larger slow cooker, mix the cranberry sauce, apricots, orange peel, orange juice, shallot, vinegar, mustard, salt, and ginger. Add the pork and spoon some of cranberry mixture on top.

Cover and cook on low for 7 to 9 hours, or until the pork is tender.

Remove the pork to a cutting board. Spoon off any fat from the top of the cranberry mixture in the slow cooker. Slice the pork into 6 thick slices. Serve topped with sauce. Garnish with the chives, if desired.

Makes 6 servings

PER SERVING: *450 calories, 32 g protein, 39 g carbohydrates, 18 g fat, 6 g saturated fat, 90 mg cholesterol, 2 g fiber, 470 mg sodium*

JERK SALMON SANDWICH

PREP TIME: 5 minutes
COOKING TIME: 8 minutes

> 2 teaspoons dry jerk seasoning (found in spice aisle of most major grocery stores)
>
> 2 boneless, skinless salmon fillets (4 ounces each)
>
> 1 tablespoon prepared horseradish
>
> ¼ cup all-fruit apricot preserves
>
> 2 whole grain hamburger buns
>
> ¼ cup watercress (optional)

Coat the grill well with olive or canola oil. Preheat to high.

Rub 1 teaspoon of the seasoning onto each fillet to cover on all sides. Place the fillets on the grill and cook for 3 to 4 minutes on each side, or until the fish is just opaque.

Meanwhile, stir the horseradish into the preserves until well combined.

About 1 minute before the salmon is cooked, place the buns, insides facing down, on the grill to toast. Remove the buns and place 1 fillet on the bottom half of each. Spoon half of the preserves mixture on top of each fillet, add the watercress, if using, and cover with the tops of the buns. Serve immediately.

Makes 2

PER SERVING: *402 calories, 30 g protein, 49 g carbohydrates, 10 g fat, 2 g saturated fat, 72 mg cholesterol, 3 g fiber, 566 mg sodium*

Note: The salmon can be made ahead of time and then wrapped in plastic wrap and refrigerated overnight. In the morning, unwrap the salmon, place on an untoasted bun, and top with the sauce. Place in a zip-top bag and refrigerate until ready to eat. (Wrap the watercress separately, if using.) To serve, remove from the bag, place between two paper plates, and microwave on low until just warm. Add the watercress and eat immediately.

Wet Your Whistle with H$_2$0

Proper hydration not only prevents you from feeling hungry (many people mistake thirst for hunger), it also can help you lose weight. In a study reported in the *Journal of Clinical Endocrinology & Metabolism*, German researchers found that after drinking 17 ounces of water, men's and women's metabolisms increased by 30 percent within a half hour. The researchers estimated that by boosting water intake by about 48 ounces—the amount in just six glasses—you could burn an extra 17,400 calories during the course of a year.

Lose 5 pounds just by drinking water? Sounds great to me! Water also helps keep you energized, improves exercise performance, and is great for your skin. I recommend buying an insulated water bottle, filling it with chilled ice water and a squeeze of lemon, and taking it with you wherever you go. Having water on hand will also help keep you from loading up on liquid calories—like soda pop.

When it comes to obesity, soda is public enemy number one. (As you'll see later, I don't believe that foods are inherently good or bad. Soda may be my sole exception. There is nothing redeeming about it.) We are literally drinking buckets of the stuff. Americans guzzle an astonishing *52 gallons* of carbonated soft drinks per person each year, according to *Beverage Digest*. Soda pop is nothing but sugar, and numerous studies show that as consumption goes up, so does weight.

Though a little orange juice in the morning is perfectly fine, too much fruit juice is a quick way to overdose on sugar, too. Eating fruit, which is filled with satisfying fiber, is always the better choice.

Other liquid calorie havens: bars, whether the coffee, alcohol, or juice variety. One large mocha latte with whipped cream packs between 500 and 800 calories. Two beers rack up 300 calories. Those fancy juice concoctions you can buy at some health clubs can easily wipe out a full workout at 300 (or more) calories each! Stick to plain old coffee; save alcohol for special occasions; and, unless you're running a marathon, drink water when you work out.

Indulge Wisely and without Guilt

There are no forbidden foods, just food choices. The goal is to make healthy food decisions about 80 percent of the time, so that you can make room for treats and less nutrient-dense fare the other 20 percent. This will help you overcome the greatest obstacle to adopting healthy eating habits—guilt. A recent survey showed that more than 75 percent of people feel guilty about eating so-called bad foods. When you attach an ethical value to food, you set up an internal battle you're bound to lose because it makes you feel deprived, angry, sad, and ultimately defeated as you give in to endless "off-limits" temptations. Listen, you're not a bad person for eating potato chips. Ice cream is not "bad." It just has a lot of calories without a whole lot of nutrition. Eat it sparingly, so you have more room for foods that deliver the daily vitamins and minerals you need without the excess fat you don't.

10-SECOND WISDOM

"Caffeine and sugar are like energy loans. They'll get you through the short term, but you end up paying it all back with interest!"

By following the 80/20 rule, you allow yourself a handful (three or four) of indulgences every month, or about one per week—enough to accommodate office parties, birthdays, and PMS cravings. The key is to not get carried away. There's an art to keeping a small indulgence from turning into a full-fledged binge. I developed this system to help my clients deviate from their healthy eating regimen without falling completely off track.

1. **Plan it.** Tell yourself you're going to have one slice of birthday cake.

2. **Pace it.** Limit treats to special occasions two or three times a month.

3. **Portion it.** Allow yourself one moderately sized serving.

4. **Enjoy it.** Pay attention to the food. Don't read or watch television.

5. **Pitch it.** Discard any leftovers to prevent temptation.

6. **Forget it.** Go right back to your healthy eating habits.

PART 2

The *Prevention's* Shortcuts Workouts

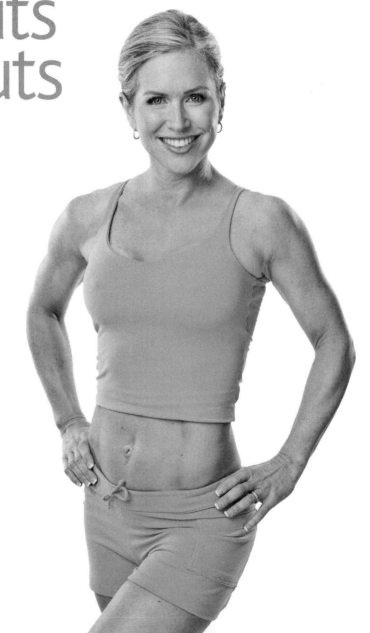

CHAPTER 4

Burn Fat with Cardio Shortcuts

Most Americans understand fuel economy very well. To save gas, you run your car less often. To save heating oil, you turn down the thermostat. The exact same strategies hold true for the energy reserves your body stores as excess fat. If you park yourself in a chair all day, you won't burn much fuel. To burn fat, you need to rev up your engine and keep your motor running as much as possible. The single best way to do that is with cardiovascular exercise. And the results of some studies suggest that the best way to do cardio exercise may be the *Prevention*'s Shortcuts way.

Inside each cell, you have hundreds or thousands of fat-burning furnaces called mitochondria. As you might expect, these cellular power plants are smaller in sedentary, unfit people, who also have fewer of them simply because they burn so little fuel that they don't need them. As you start exercising, however, your body gets the signal that it needs to ramp up production, improve its facilities to burn more fat, and power your muscles. As a result, it beefs up the size of your mitochondria by up to 35 percent and increases the number of these fat-burning furnaces by 15 percent. In short, by doing regular aerobic exercise, you can literally turn your body into a fat-burning machine. That's not all (though admittedly, it's mainly what most women I know care about!). Decades of research confirms that regular cardiovascular (or aerobic) exercise:

- **Strengthens your heart.** Walking just 1 hour a week slices your risk of having a heart attack in half. On the *Prevention*'s Shortcuts program, you'll do one 10-minute cardio walking workout each day, with a second one 3 to 5 days a

1-MINUTE WONDER
TAP YOUR TOES!

Studies show fidgeters burn about 200 to 500 more calories every day than nonfidgeters—that's the equivalent of a 30- to 40-minute workout! Even if you're tied to your desk all day, bounce your knees up and down and change positions frequently. Every little bit of movement increases your body's demand for oxygen and burns calories.

week. That's a total of at least 1 hour 40 minutes of walking per week. Your heart thanks you!

- **Keeps your arteries clear.** Studies show that physical activity is inversely related to the progressive buildup of plaque in the carotid artery leading to the heart. Research also indicates that for lowering triglycerides, a type of blood fat that raises heart attack risk, accumulated 10-minute bursts of exercise like the *Prevention's* Shortcuts program are more effective than longer, continuous cardio workouts.

- **Increases your lung capacity.** The *Prevention's* Shortcuts cardio program may even improve your cardio health twice as fast as other programs, since research shows that shorter bouts of exercise can increase maximal oxygen consumption (a measure of lung, heart, and muscle strength) by nearly twice as much as 30-minute workouts.

- **Reduces your risk of diabetes.** Research shows that regular exercise can improve your insulin sensitivity (a measure of how efficiently your body stimulates glucose, or blood sugar, metabolism) by about 24 percent.

- **Beats the blues.** Mental health studies show that exercise can work as well as drugs for lifting depression and easing anxiety. Exercise endorphins are like "happy drugs." And they're much cheaper than therapy!

If you could put all those benefits in a pill, it would fly off the pharmacy shelves faster than drug companies could manufacture it. That's the beauty of the *Prevention's* Shortcuts program. The only prescription you need is this book. And the only side effects are weight loss, disease protection, and a longer, happier life!

FOLLOW YOUR HEART

Doing a *Prevention*'s Shortcuts cardio workout is as easy as walking around your neighborhood. But if you really want to burn fat and make the most out of every active minute, you need to be sure you're working at just the right intensity, which means monitoring your heart rate.

LIFESTYLE SHORTCUT
WALK THIS WAY

The amount of time Americans spend walking has dropped 42 percent during the past 20 years. The number of obese and overweight men and women has increased by 40 percent over the same 2 decades. Some quick ways to walk more:

- Walk with co-workers to brainstorm instead of sitting in a conference room. (You can even have a code phrase, like "Let's walk," that you can e-mail to your colleagues when you have some important news to share.)

- Instead of driving around town to run errands, park at a central location and walk to each destination.

- Enter the mall at the farthest entrance from your favorite store so you have to walk the entire length of the shopping center before you can get to your destination.

- When a bad spell at work has you craving chips or candy, take 2 minutes to walk off your frustration instead of hitting the vending machine.

- When you talk on the phone, walk around instead of sitting in a chair.

- Take the stairs no matter where you are. (I play a little game with myself—I won't let myself use the escalator unless I have a heavy suitcase with me.)

- On rainy or snowy days, use an indoor walking or cardio video. When you have breaks in your day, you can do a quick 10-minute portion to get your heart pumping.

- Practice moving meditation. Use walking as a time to quiet your mind and organize your thoughts. Try walking a few blocks each night after dinner. Reflect on the day. Work through issues that are nagging at you. And take a few moments to feel thankful for your life.

When you exercise, your heart has to beat faster to pump more oxygen-rich blood and nutrients to your working muscles. The harder you work, the faster your heart beats. You can measure precisely how many times your heart is beating per minute by using a heart rate monitor, a transmitter that straps around your chest at your bra line. It picks up the electrical signal sent from your beating heart and transmits that information (wirelessly) to a special watch you wear on your wrist so you can easily read your bpm (beats per minute) at any time during your workout. Most models let you program your exercising heart rate range into the watch, and it beeps at you if you fall below or push above your target exercise zone. I consider mine my cardiovascular dashboard—full of feedback and data to keep me motivated. I have a beautiful diamond-studded watch I *could* wear, but I'm so addicted to my monitor, I only take it off and switch watches if I'm going somewhere *really* fancy!

The *Prevention's* Shortcuts cardio workouts require you to exercise within an aerobic heart range where your body is working hard enough to reap benefits but not so hard that you run the risk of burning out or hurting yourself. This target heart rate range is based on your maximum heart rate—the most beats per minute your heart can pump out—which is determined mostly by genetics. Below is the simplest formula for figuring out your maximum heart rate and target heart rate. (This formula is not exact but helps you get started. The booklet that comes with your heart rate monitor will explain other formulas you can use along with the monitor to figure your target heart rate.)

1. Subtract your age from 220 (i.e., 220 – 45 years = 175); this is your maximum heart rate in beats per minute.

2. Calculate 65 percent of your maximum heart rate (i.e., 175 × 0.65 = 113); this is the low end of your target heart rate range.

3. Calculate 85 percent of your maximum heart rate (i.e., 175 × 0.85 = 148); this is the high end of your target heart rate range.

Using this formula, a 45-year-old woman should try to keep her heart rate between 113 and 148 during exercise. It's important to remember that this formula is only a guideline. If you are already pretty fit, you may find that your target heart rate feels too easy, in which case, add 5 to 10 beats to the low- and high-end numbers and see if it feels better.

No heart rate monitor? Use the rate of perceived exertion (RPE) scale instead. Monitoring your exercise effort by rating your perceived exertion is a fancy way of saying that you're listening to your body. It's a 1-to-10 scale that allows you to judge your effort based on how you're feeling.

0–1 Chilling out on the recliner, watching Animal Planet. You're barely moving and lifting nothing heavier than the remote.

2–3 Meandering through Disney World. You're moving, but it's minimal effort, like strolling or stretching. Easy and slow.

4–5 Brisk walking, easy hiking, cycling on a flat road. You're breaking a light sweat and your muscles are warm, but you can still talk easily enough to hold a conversation.

6–7 Power walking. You're moving and working hard enough to be breathing faster. You couldn't have a rambling conversation, but you can utter a sentence or two without gasping.

8–9 Jogging or walking as fast as your feet will carry you. You're huffing and puffing and can speak only a few words at a time.

10   Sprinting or another all-out effort. You may only be able to sustain this effort for 15 to 60 seconds. No speaking, just heavy breathing.

Studies show that if you use RPE carefully and consistently, it can be just as good as heart rate monitoring. Personally, I think the two work best together. I find that if you tend to let your mind wander during workouts, RPE isn't as effective as having a monitor that reminds you to pick up the pace or—this happens less often—slow down. If you use RPE, you're going to need to be a mindful exerciser—no watching *Law & Order* reruns or reading magazines (though music may help). Pay attention to your effort and stay in the zone.

The closer you get to 10 on the RPE scale, the more calories you burn per minute. Since level 10 is *so* intense, however, you can't sustain it for very many seconds, let alone minutes. Most of the *Prevention*'s Shortcuts cardio workouts will keep your perceived exertion between a 6 and a 9, where your calorie burn is high but you also can sustain the effort.

THE FAT-BURNING MYTH

About 10 or 15 years ago, some exercise scientists suggested that women who wanted to burn more of their fat stores (rather than burning stored carbs) should keep their heart rates low and work out in a so-called fat-burning zone. This was a case of good science gone bad. I still get questions today from women who say they don't want to work too hard because they're trying to burn fat.

Here's the deal. Conventional wisdom says that low-intensity exercise—below 65 percent of your maximum heart rate or about 3 to 4 on the RPE scale—burns 60 percent of calories from fat, while higher intensities burn only about 35 percent of calories as fat. But the important component most people don't take into account is how many *calories* low-intensity exercise burns versus how many high intensity burns. If a 140-pound woman walks for 10 minutes at a low to moderate intensity, she'll burn about 40 calories, 24 of them from fat (the rest from carbs). If that same woman breaks out into a 5-mph jog for the same amount of time, she'll burn about 85 calories, 30 of them as fat. So in the end, when the woman exercised harder, she not only burned more calories, which is the only way you lose weight, but also burned a greater amount of fat. That's why the *Prevention's* Shortcuts cardio workouts make you increase your perceived exertion to between 6 and 9 or keep your heart rate in the 65 to 85 percent range, preferably on the higher end as you become more fit.

Upping your intensity also gives you what I call a bonus burn. The more oxygen and calories you use while you exercise, the more your body will continue to use

LIFESTYLE SHORTCUT
TAKE IT OUTSIDE!

I'm a big fan of outdoor exercise whenever possible. The treadmill is a lifesaver for me in Minnesota when the mercury is just a sliver of red at the bottom of the thermometer, but nothing beats the great outdoors for energizing every cell and boosting your mood. It's a chemical fact. Australian researchers have found that men and women who run outdoors have even higher levels of feel-good endorphins afterward than their treadmill-running peers.

when you're done. The easiest way to use more oxygen and calories is to up your intensity. One recent study showed that women working out at a high intensity continued to burn nearly *twice* as many calories 3 hours after they wrapped up their workout as those who worked out at a low intensity. That's why my Need for Speed (page 85) and Fast and Focused (page 86) workouts are high energy (yet completely manageable for every woman)—so you get a big bonus burn after every effort.

The bottom line is that with Prevention's Shortcuts cardio walking workouts, you'll be working out at an intensity that is comfortably hard. For some people, that may be running on a track; for others, just walking around the block. You'll know you're in the right zone if you have to drop your jaw and breathe through your mouth. If you can still breathe through your nose, you're not working hard enough to burn measurable calories and lose fat.

JOYFUL MOVEMENT

Not a week goes by without someone asking me what the "best" kind of cardio-vascular activity is. Should they run? Ride a bike? Use a stairclimber or elliptical trainer? My answer is always the same: The best kind of cardio activity for you is whatever you will do! It's true that, minute for minute, running probably burns the most calories of any aerobic exercise (except maybe jumping rope), but running is not for everyone. And if you hate it, you'll never do it. That's why I've built the *Prevention*'s Shortcuts cardio program around an activity that millions of American women do every day, without a second thought: walking.

Human beings are born to walk. The moment our legs are strong enough, we pull ourselves up from a crawl and teeter around until we master locomotion—and then we're off! Walking strengthens your heart and lungs, lubricates your joints, builds your bones, and gets you where you want to go. What's more, walking works for weight loss. Done briskly, it can burn almost as many calories as jogging. And it's easier on your joints, especially if you're overweight.

To get the biggest calorie burn from every step, walk briskly, purposefully, and,

10-SECOND WISDOM

"Walking helps me stay fit because you can do it anytime, anywhere. I sneak extra activity into my life by parking far away from where I'm going, riding my bike to do errands instead of driving, and finding reasons to make multiple trips up and down the stairs."

Donna, 43

most important, with good form. When you walk with proper form, you use more muscles in your upper body and core, so you use more energy. You also activate more muscles in your hips, butt, and thighs, so you tone and shape those areas as you move along. What's more, walking will feel easier. Good technique means less wear and tear on your knees, ankles, and hips, so you're less likely to injure yourself or have to stop because of achy joints.

Here is a head-to-toe look at proper walking form.

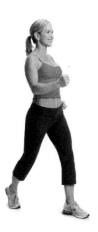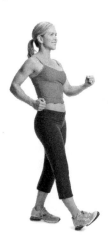

Head: Hold your head high and lift your chin so your eyes are looking straight ahead. Picture a string attached to the crown of your head, holding it straight up, so your ears fall directly over your shoulders.

Shoulders: Roll your shoulders up and then let them fall down and back in a natural, open position. Maintain that posture, not allowing them to creep up toward your ears.

Chest: Keep your breastbone lifted so your lungs can fully inflate with fresh oxygen for your working muscles.

Arms: Bend your elbows about 90 degrees, close your hands into loose fists, and pump your arms forward and back as you walk.

Abdominals: "Zip" up your abs by contracting them and pulling your navel toward your spine as though you were snapping a snug pair of pants. Keep your abs engaged as you walk.

Back: Walk tall by keeping your back straight. Avoid slumping forward or arching back.

Knees: Keep your knees soft. Don't lock or hyperextend them.

Feet: With each stride, plant your heel and roll onto the ball of your foot, pushing off forcefully with your toes to take quick, smooth steps. Your feet should feel stable as they strike the ground. If they seem to be rolling inward or outward, you may need new walking shoes. Most shoe companies make "motion control" shoes for people with particularly high or low arches, to avoid too much side-to-side foot motion that can strain your ankles, knees, and hips.

Before you read any farther, I want you to stop right here and commit yourself to doing one of the workouts in this chapter *today* (or tomorrow, at the latest, if you're reading this late at night). Put it on your calendar and do it. Do the same thing tomorrow and the day after that, until it becomes a habit.

So now you've made your promise to me. And here's my promise to you: Once you try the *Prevention*'s Shortcuts interval workouts, you're going to catch the "cardio bug." No one ever believes it. But it happens every time. You do your 10 minutes, and it feels good and you think, "Well, what if I did 10 minutes more . . . ?" Soon you're doing a second *Prevention*'s Shortcuts workout, and you're burning more calories and feeling better. So then you decide to do three *Prevention*'s Shortcuts during the day. Cardio has an addictive side to it. You feel euphoric and get so hooked on the mood improvement and self-confidence boost that you want to do more. I can't tell you the number of adults who run up to me like kids brimming with excitement, proudly declaring, "I'm going to walk a 5-K!" "I'm going to walk a half-marathon!" It's the snowball effect. You just have to get that ball rolling!

Naturally, if you've been sedentary for a long time, it may still take you 6 to 8 weeks to get into the exercise habit, no matter how good it feels. So be patient with yourself. Keep a chart. Journal your progress, and read it every day. Give yourself credit for every little gain. And remember to *have fun!*

NO TIME? NO PROBLEM

When it comes to moving your body, more is always better. So by all means, take a good 30-minute walk whenever time allows. But remember, it's cumulative time that counts. Life *does* get crazy sometimes. Too many women make the mistake of thinking that if they can't get at least 20 or 30 minutes in, they may as well not bother. In fact, studies show that people who do absolutely no exercise for 2 weeks lose much more fitness than people who do even just a little something every day. The body adapts to what you do. So move it daily! Taking an all-or-nothing approach is the surest way to derail your fitness goals.

The trick is to follow the *Prevention's* Shortcuts program and use whatever time you have to your best advantage. That means doing things you already know how to do: walking more often, taking the stairs, standing up now and then to stretch and move around, and so on. But, of course, you need more than that. As I explained in the previous chapters, the best way for busy people to get their prescribed daily dose of exercise is to do several *Prevention's* Shortcuts workouts throughout the day. Again, the key to these workouts is that they make you crank up the intensity and work harder than usual. That means increasing your perceived exertion to between 6 and 9 or keeping your heart rate in the 65 to 85 percent range, preferably on the higher end as you become more fit.

Here are my favorite short-burst workouts that can fry lots of fat when time is tight. You can do them around the block, on your favorite walking trail, or indoors on the treadmill.

10-SECOND WISDOM

"If you're creative, you can make any activity more active. I do situps and pushups while my daughter is playing on the floor; I do calf raises while in line at the grocery store; I throw in a block or two of jogging while pushing the stroller around the neighborhood. There's always something you can do to make sure you don't miss working out."

Katherine, 29

CARDIO WALKING WORKOUTS

Ready. Set. Let's burn some calories! The following mini walking workouts will burn about 100 calories a pop and are guaranteed to set your fat-burning thermostat on high after you're done. Every day, do at least one of them. Three to 5 days a week, do a second one. Following this *Prevention's* Shortcuts program of 10-minute interval workouts can improve your endurance as much as you would by doing slower-paced aerobic exercise for hours each week. Researchers have found that people who did four 30-second sprints (with 4 minutes of rest between efforts) on stationary bikes three times a week reaped identical fitness gains to those who pedaled for *2 hours* at a moderate pace three times a week.

You can do these workouts inside or out. If you're inside on the treadmill, turn up the intensity by increasing your speed or incline while pumping your arms. If walking outdoors, increase intensity by taking shorter, quicker strides and strong arm pumps to achieve the appropriate RPE goals.

Important note: The brevity of these *Prevention's* Shortcuts workouts does not give you license to blow off your warmup and cooldown. It's important to warm your muscles and connective tissues before pushing them with more intense exercise. The best way to do that is to walk at a lower intensity for a couple of minutes before ramping up the exertion. Simply take the first minute to walk at a slow pace and get your blood flowing. After you've done the workout, finish up with a cooldown, just slowing the pace or lowering the intensity for a minute or two, to help your heart rate gradually return to normal. Then take the time to stretch the muscles you just worked, using the flexibility exercises that start on page 300.

Quick Calorie Burners

These workouts are designed to burn calories at a quicker pace than your normal walking workout. So when you're pressed for time, you can trade off intensity for duration.

Need for Speed

MINUTE	ACTIVITY	RPE
1	Warmup walk/walk in place	Achieve 4
2	Moderate-pace walk	4–5
3	Brisk walk	6–7
4	Fast, hard walk/pump arms	8–9
5	Fast, hard walk/pump arms	8–9
6	Moderate walk	4–5
7	Brisk walk	6–7
8	Fast, hard walk/pump arms	8–9
9	Fast, hard walk/pump arms	8–9
10	Slowly cool down	4

Fast and Focused

MINUTE	ACTIVITY	RPE
1	Warmup walk/walk in place	Achieve 4
2	Moderate-pace walk	4–5
3	Brisk pace, pumping arms	8–9
4	Fast, almost breathless by end	9–10
5	Moderate-pace walk	4–5
6	Brisk pace, pumping arms	8–9
7	Fast, almost breathless by end	9–10
8	Brisk pace, pumping arms	8–9
9	Fast, almost breathless	9–10
10	Moderate to cooldown pace	5

Fat-Sizzling Walking Workouts

Both of these are great for days when you need to blow out the cobwebs and burn calories but want to move at a more comfortable pace. They can easily be extended to go a little longer when time permits.

Strong and Steady

MINUTE	ACTIVITY	RPE
1	Warmup walk/walk in place	Achieve 4
2	Moderate-pace walk	5
3	Moderate-pace walk	5
4	Pick up the pace	6
5	Pick up the pace	6
6	Pick up the pace	6
7	Brisk but not breathless: power-walk pace	7
8	Brisk but not breathless: power-walk pace	7
9	Brisk but not breathless: power-walk pace	7
10	Moderate to cooldown pace	4–5

Pyramid Power

This is like a good hiking workout—you hike up the hill and back down. It's a great way to combat boredom. Climb up to a good pace, and then come down on the other side.

MINUTE	ACTIVITY	RPE
1	Warmup walk/walk in place	Achieve 4
2	Moderate-pace walk	5
3	Pick up the pace	6
4	Brisk but not breathless	7–8
5	Brisk, almost breathless: Work it!	9–10
6	Brisk, almost breathless; back off ever so slightly	8–9
7	Brisk but not breathless	7–8
8	Begin to slow a bit	6
9	Moderate-pace walk	5
10	Moderate to cooldown pace	4

Bun Burners

Both these workouts use the incline feature on your treadmill. Hitting the hills is a great way to increase intensity, since engaging large muscle groups—like the quads, hamstrings, and glutes—gets your heart pumping quickly to burn calories faster. Incline workouts are a fun change, and, best of all, you can't beat them for shaping your buns.

Rolling Hills

Beginners, slow mph to 3; advanced, raise to 5 to achieve correct RPE.

MINUTE	SPEED	INCLINE	RPE
1	Get to 4	1	2–3
2	4	2–3	3–4
3	4	4–6	6–7
4	4	8	8–9
5	4	4–6	4–7
6	4	8	8–9

(continued)

Rolling Hills *(continued)*

MINUTE	SPEED	INCLINE	RPE
7	4	4–6	6–7
8	4	8	8–9
9	4	2–3	4–5
10	Back down	1	2–3

Conquer the Mountain

This one's a little harder; it picks up to a jogging pace as you go up and over each hill at 6 mph.

MINUTE	SPEED	INCLINE	RPE
1	Get to 4	1	2–3
2	4.5	3	4–5
3	6	5	8–9
4	4.5	1	4–5
5	4.5	3	6–7
6	6	5	8–9
7	4.5	1	4–5
8	4.5	3	6–7
9	6	5	8–9
10	Back down	1	2–3

10 CARDIO QUICK TAKES

Think you can't boost your fitness 1 minute at a time? Here are 10 high-energy exercises that will make you think again! In Chapters 6 and 10, you'll find these interspersed with strength exercises to create *Prevention*'s Shortcuts to busting through weight loss plateaus. These moves are especially ideal when you're having one of those days where you just can't catch a break. Sprinkle them throughout your day to boost your energy and keep your metabolism on high. Just remember your better-than-nothing attitude, pick one of these moves, and go! Everyone can spare a minute.

POWER JAB DRILL

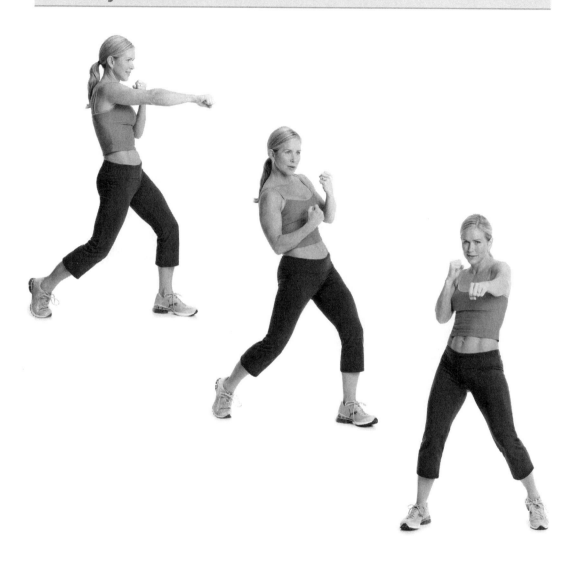

Try shadowboxing. Stand in front of a mirror and do your best Rocky imitation, throwing strong punches, short jabs, and uppercuts.

POWER MARCH

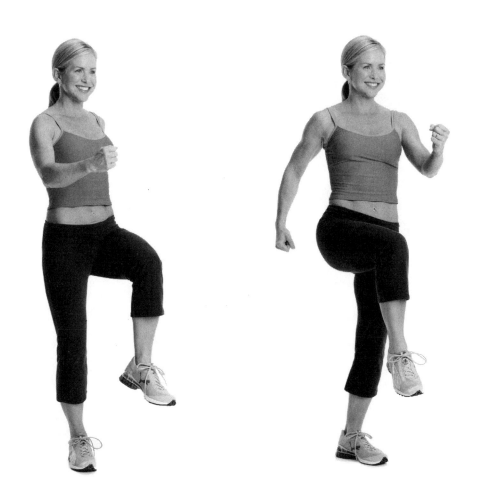

March in place, lifting your knees high as you pump your arms to get your heart rate up.

SKI HOP

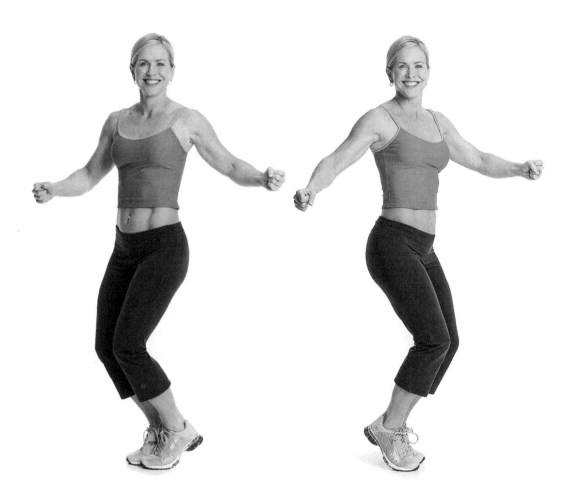

With your feet together, jump from side to side, landing with your knees bent. The wider you jump and the lower you squat into the jump, the harder you'll work.

SPEED SKATING

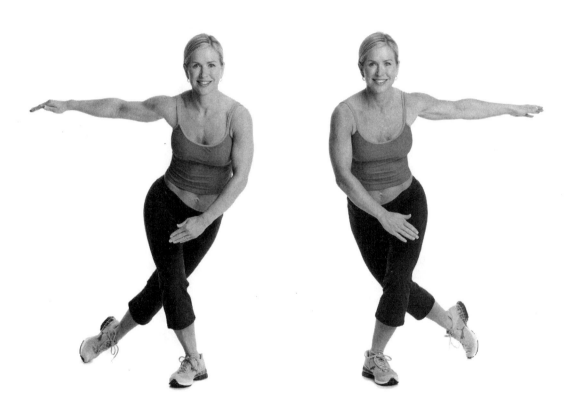

Starting with your feet together, bend your knees and, with your right leg, jump to your right, keeping your body low and landing with a bent right knee. Immediately sweep your left foot behind your right ankle, push off, and jump to your left.

BASKETBALL JUMP SHOT

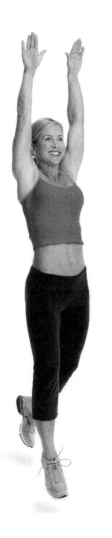 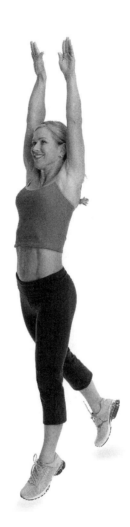

Pretend to shoot some hoops. Step forward on one foot and hop up into the air as if to dunk a basketball. Alternate feet, stepping and hopping. You can step up onto a step to add intensity.

STAIR BLASTER

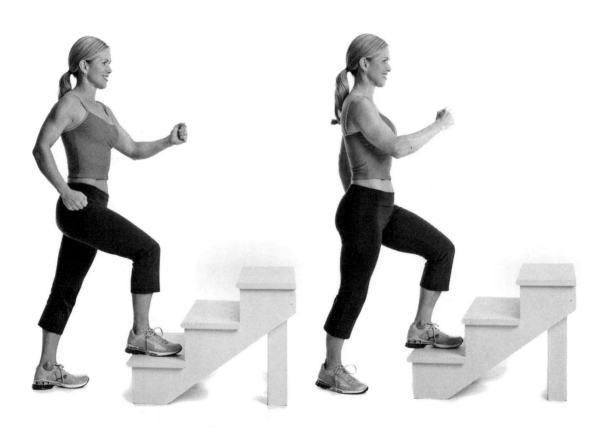

Stand facing a step. Briskly step up with your right and left foot and then down with your right and left foot.

SQUAT HOP

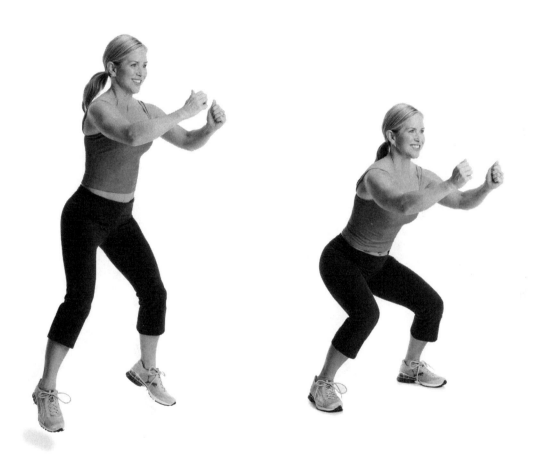

Stand with your feet wide. Lower into a squat and hop forward four times, keeping your feet wide and your legs bent into a squat. Walk back and repeat.

SPLIT JUMP

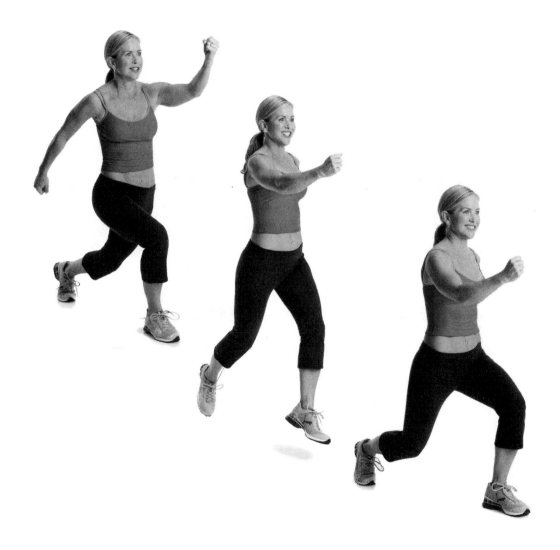

Begin in the basic lunge position. Leap straight up and switch legs in the air, landing with bent knees into a lunge with the opposite leg in front.

LIGHTING THE TORCH

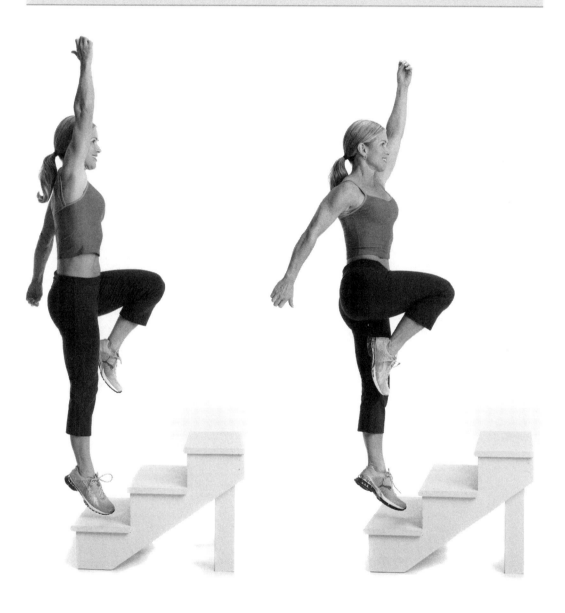

Stand on the floor in front of a staircase, and step onto the bottom step with your right foot while simultaneously lifting your left knee and right arm. Step back down to the floor with your left foot and then your right, then immediately step up with your left foot while raising your right knee and left arm.

TIRE DRILL

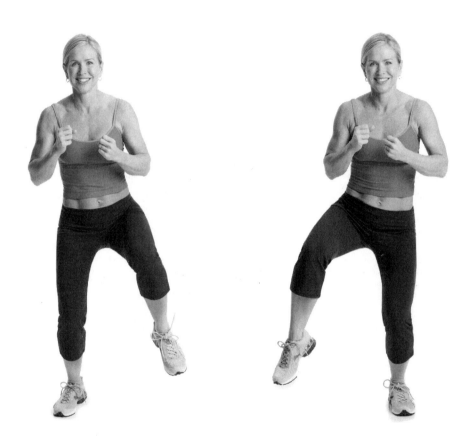

Standing with your feet wide apart and your knees bent about 45 degrees, lift one knee and then the other, taking short quick steps forward as though you were running through tires.

STRETCH IT OUT

Flexibility is key to maintaining your range of motion and enjoying physical activity through your whole life. The best time to stretch is after cooling down from a cardio workout, while your muscles are still warm. Stretching helps to relax and lengthen your muscles, so you're less likely to be stiff and sore after a good hard effort. It also improves flexibility in your joints and helps reduce your risk of overuse injuries like tendinitis and plantar fasciitis (heel pain).

Beginning on the next page, you'll find my top-10 essential stretches. These moves take you through all the major muscle groups, giving them the treatment they deserve. Hold each stretch for 20 to 30 seconds.

1-MINUTE WONDER
DO "INVISIBLE" EXERCISE

Often, what the world can't see you doing is more important than what it can see. Those are words spoken by many a Pilates instructor. Practice contracting your transversus abdominis (i.e., "scooping your abs" as described on page 194) for 1 minute while in the car, on the subway, checking out at the grocery store, or even lying in bed. I give this advice to my new students as their first step for mastering flat abs. A few weeks ago, I saw a woman from one of my classes in the grocery store. She walked by, smiling, and said, "I'm doing it." And I thought, "You sure are!"

IT BAND FORWARD BEND

TARGETS HIPS AND GLUTES

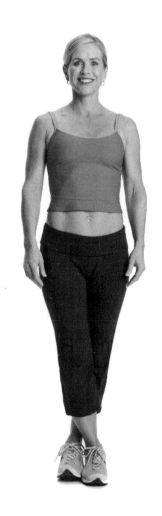
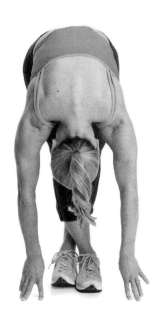

Stand with your right leg crossed in front of your left.

Bend down toward your toes as far as comfortably possible. Walk your hands toward your right foot to deepen the stretch in your IT band (iliotibial band—a band of connective tissue that runs from your hip, along your thigh, down to the outside of your knee). Return to the starting position. Repeat to the opposite side.

RUNNER'S STRETCH

TARGETS HIP FLEXORS

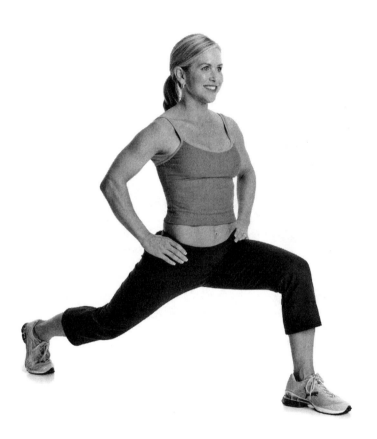

Stand in a lunge position, keeping your front knee above the ankle and balancing on your back toe (or drop your back knee to the floor). Gently press your back hip toward the floor, lengthening the hip flexor muscles. Hold, and then repeat on the other side.

SIDE-LYING QUAD STRETCH

TARGETS QUADRICEPS

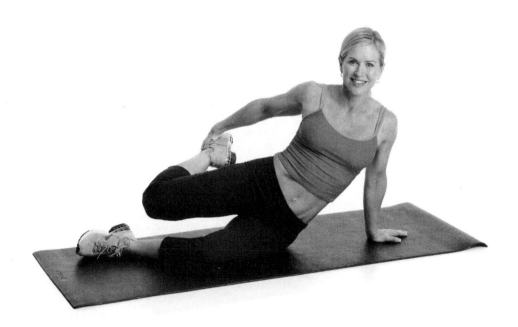

Sit on your left hip with your legs extended to your right, knees slightly bent. Place your left hand on the floor, in line with your left shoulder, for support. Reach behind you with your right hand and grasp your right ankle and gently pull your heel toward your glutes, keeping your hip pressed against the floor. Repeat on the opposite side.

LYING SPINAL TWIST

TARGETS BACK, TORSO, HIPS, AND SHOULDERS

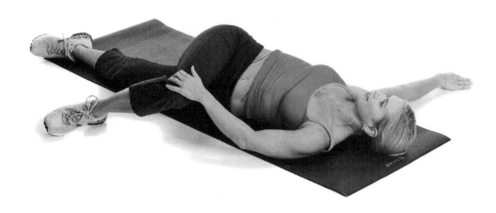

Lie faceup on the floor with your legs straight and your arms extended out to the sides. Bring your right knee in toward your chest. Grasping the outside of your right knee with your left hand, gently rotate your hips and pull your knee toward the floor. Try to keep your shoulders on the floor. Switch sides.

SEATED STRADDLE REACH

TARGETS HAMSTRINGS, INNER THIGHS, AND LOWER BACK

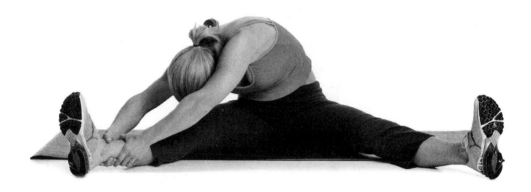

Sit on the floor with your back straight and your legs spread as wide as possible. Keeping your back straight, gently bend at your hips and lean forward over one leg as far as comfortably possible, keeping both legs straight. Bend your knees to modify for tight hamstrings. Repeat on the opposite side.

CALF STRETCH

TARGETS CALVES AND ACHILLES TENDONS

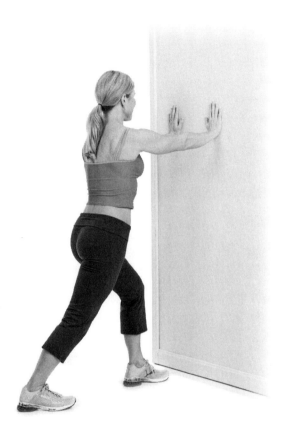

Stand at arm's length from a wall, facing it. Place your right foot behind your left, keeping both heels flat on the floor. Lean toward the wall, slightly bending your knees until you feel the stretch up the backs of your heels and calves, especially in your right leg. Switch feet and repeat.

This stretch is especially useful after any cardio exercise that requires jumping, lunging, or hill climbing.

DOOR CHEST STRETCH

TARGETS PECTORALS AND FRONT SHOULDERS

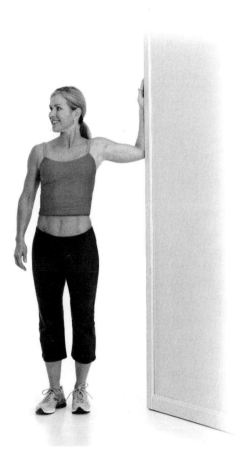

Stand in a doorway. Lift your left arm out and bend it at the elbow so your upper arm is parallel to the floor and your fingers are pointed toward the ceiling. Press your hand and forearm against the door frame. Rotate your body toward the right, causing your left arm to be pulled back so you feel the stretch across your chest and shoulder. Repeat with your right arm.

C-CURVE STRETCH

TARGETS ENTIRE BACK AND REAR SHOULDERS

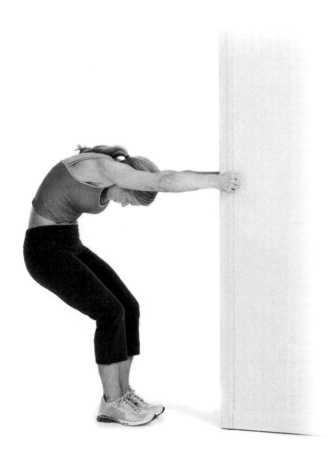

Standing an arm's length away from a door frame, a pillar, or a tree, position your feet hip-width apart and grip the door frame at shoulder height. Slightly bend your knees and create a curve with your back. Round your spine from the nape of your neck to your tailbone, and slightly pull away from the door frame.

OVERHEAD TRICEPS STRETCH

TARGETS TRICEPS

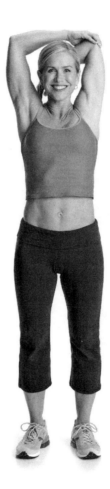

Stand with your feet shoulder-width apart and your back straight. Raise your left arm up over your head, bend your elbow, and reach your hand down behind your head to the middle of your back. The fingers of your left hand should fall between your shoulder blades, and your left elbow should point toward the ceiling. Keeping your shoulders down, grasp your left elbow with your right hand and gently push the elbow down until you feel the stretch in the back of your left arm. Repeat with the right arm.

FOLDOVER CHEST EXPANSION

TARGETS HAMSTRINGS, SHOULDERS, AND CHEST

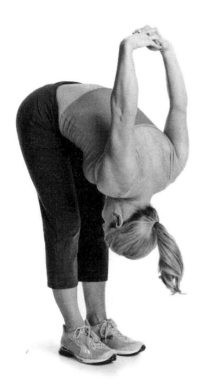

Stand with your feet shoulder-width apart, knees slightly bent. Interlace your fingers behind your back (or hold the end of a towel if your shoulders are tight). Push your chest forward, keeping your spine long, as you fold over into a forward bend. Drop your forehead toward your knees and lift your arms up toward your upper back.

CHAPTER 5

Big Weight Loss

If you have 25 or more pounds to lose, you've likely already tried a ton of weight loss tricks. Maybe you've even reached your goal weight a few times, only to see the excess pounds come cascading back just a few months later. Don't be too hard on yourself. We've been tricked into believing that fad diets (grapefruit for breakfast, lunch, and dinner, anyone?), prescription drugs (remember the Fen-Phen debacle?), and herbal potions like "carb blockers" or, worse, ephedra (nature's speed) will help us be suddenly slim.

The real deal is this: Most women gain weight through small "nickel and dime" lifestyle choices—like ordering nachos with dinner and driving down the block instead of walking—that add up over time. Starting in your thirties, as your hormones change and you have to devote more time to sedentary activities like work and driving kids around, you begin to lose ½ to 1 pound of muscle a year. Sounds like you should be getting skinnier, right? Unfortunately, that's not how it works. As your muscle mass diminishes, your metabolism slows down to the tune of 1 percent for every pound of muscle loss. So your percentage of body fat increases—even if you're not eating one morsel more.

As if the metabolism meltdown and midlife spread weren't bad enough, diminished muscle mass makes life harder. Carrying groceries, lugging laundry, even fun stuff like running around in the yard with your dog are all more difficult. Heck, without strong core and back muscles, just standing up straight can feel like a chore. So guess what? As daily life gets harder, you move less . . . and gain more.

The good news is that stepping off this slippery slope is a snap. The *Prevention's* Shortcuts program is ideal for women with lots of weight to lose because it doesn't demand you change everything in your life in one fell swoop. Rather, it slims you down the same way you put on the weight—one little step at a time. And as we explained in Chapter 1, research shows that by using the *Prevention's* Shortcuts approach, you may lose as much as 30 percent more weight than you would with traditional, longer workouts. Better yet, you'll maintain your weight loss better than with other programs, particularly if you follow Lifestyle Shortcuts, like the one at the end of the chapter.

LIFT WEIGHT TO LOSE WEIGHT

Strength training is the single best way to fire up a sluggish metabolism. Lifting weights for just 10 minutes a day can make a dramatic difference in the way you look and feel. Why? Because it restores the youthful muscle tone you've lost over time. Research shows that if you work every major muscle group twice a week—as you will with the *Prevention's* Shortcuts system—you can replace 2 pounds of lost muscle in as little as 8 weeks. That's 5 to 10 years' worth of metabolism-revving lean tissue in 2 months.

In one study, women who started strength training were able to boost their resting metabolism, or the number of calories you burn when you're just hanging around, by 7 percent, or 88 calories a day. Metabolism researchers say you can expect to burn about an additional 15 calories for every pound of active muscle tissue you replace. Those extra calories combined with your workout burn and post-exercise burn mean that in just 16 weeks, you could fry an additional 200 calories (enough to burn off a glazed doughnut). May not sound like much, but it's enough to burn off 9 pounds in a year! And that doesn't count the calories you burn while doing all the other activities you start to enjoy because you have the strength and energy to do them—playing a singles tennis match instead of doubles, gardening all day long, playing kickball with your kids or grandkids, trying a new circuit class at the health club, or finally joining your neighborhood group of power walkers! You'll burn more because you'll be more active all day, every day.

So why don't more women strength train? It just doesn't occur to most women—and that's something I'm here to change. Others can't shake the old fear that weights will make them look masculine. To those women I ask, "Do Jennifer Aniston, Cindy

Crawford, Angelina Jolie, or Heidi Klum look like men to you?" All those gorgeous, shapely, lean women gracing the covers of magazines lift weights to look that way. The *Prevention's* Shortcuts dumbbell workouts will help you look smaller, not bigger. Yes, you will gain muscle. But remember, a pound of muscle is more compact (and looks better) than a larger, lumpy pound of fat. And as far as getting bulky, forget it. All women produce some "male" hormones like testosterone, but far less than men, so you won't grow bulging biceps like the "governator." What you *will* do is tighten up those notoriously flabby spots on your hips, butt, thighs, and upper arms. You'll also get stronger—30 to 50 percent stronger, according to exercise physiologists. That means you can walk faster, play with the dog longer, and look and feel more like you did when you were in your twenties.

And that's not all. Reams of research collected over the past decade have proven that resistance training reduces your risk of heart disease, diabetes, obesity, and even

"E-WHAT?"

Women often prefer cardio to weight training because they believe cardio is the only way to burn lots of calories and shed fat. What they fail to realize is that pumping iron gives you a greater calorie burn after you're done. The scientific term is excess postexercise oxygen consumption, or EPOC. The more oxygen your body uses, the more calories you burn. And after strength training, your muscles need plenty of O_2 to rebuild, repair, and grow stronger and more toned.

In one study, exercise researchers from Shippensburg University in Pennsylvania had women either exercise on a treadmill or perform strength training exercises to burn the same

number of calories, then measured the women's EPOC to see how many calories they continued to burn after they were done. You guessed it: EPOC was significantly higher in the resistance training group for 30 minutes after exercise, yielding a bigger fat-burning bang for their exercise time.

What's more, muscle tissue is more metabolically active than fat, so the more lean muscle tissue you build, the more oxygen your body uses (and the more calories you burn) all day long— even while you're sleeping. Burning fat while you sleep? Now that's worth picking up some weights for.

depression. It's also the best way to build bones. When researchers asked 37 women to lift weights just twice a week for 16 weeks, they improved their bone density by 50 percent.

For women who have 25-plus pounds to lose, I've specially tailored the program to target all the major muscle groups in the body to build maximum lean muscle tissue, which will be actively burning calories in your body at all times, whether at play or at rest. If you belong to a gym, you can do all these exercises there, but you can also perform them right in the comfort of your own living room. All you need is a few hand weights (dumbbells) and a mat or carpeted floor.

> **10-SECOND WISDOM**
> "Life is like a bike—in order to stay balanced, you have to keep moving!"

Though it's natural to feel excited as you embark on a new exercise program, I encourage you to ease into the *Prevention*'s Shortcuts exercises. If you're new to strength training, your body isn't used to using your muscles in such an intense way. I hate the thought of anyone hobbling around the house for days after a workout because of sore muscles! Use the first few sessions to familiarize yourself with the moves and learn proper form. Once you feel comfortable with your technique, add a little more weight and start to push yourself. It may be a slower start than you'd envisioned, but you'll be more likely to stick to it and get great results.

Each workout should take just 10 minutes, give or take a few seconds. That's allowing for the time it takes to switch positions for each new exercise, grab a heavier or lighter set of hand weights, swallow a sip of water, etc. It does not, however, allow for interruptions such as answering the phone, changing a diaper, or emptying the dishwasher. As much as possible, try to stay focused on your workout for the full 10 consecutive minutes. Your body will thank you.

Do one workout from this chapter 3 to 5 days a week. If you feel highly motivated or have extra time, you can do more than one workout in a day, but that's not necessary. I've provided three different Big Weight Loss workouts—A, B, and C—and you can choose whichever one(s) you like, though I recommend mixing them up rather than doing the same one every time. I also recommend plenty of cardio—at least one of the Chapter 4 workouts every day, plus a second one of those workouts 3 to 5 days a week. And whenever possible, try a Lifestyle Shortcut, a 1-Minute Wonder, or any of the *Prevention*'s Shortcuts workouts from any other chapters in the book that strike

SMART STRENGTH TRAINING

To get the most out of strength training, proper technique is essential. The following tips will make your efforts more effective and safer.

Get the blood flowing. You don't need a lengthy warmup. But take a minute or two to jog in place or do a few jumping jacks to increase your circulation and warm up your muscles and connective tissue, so they're less likely to get strained when you do your first move.

Go slow. Unless you're doing one of my plyometric exercises (quick jumping or hopping moves), always lift slowly. It helps you maintain proper form. You'll activate more muscle fibers when you move purposely through your full range of motion than if you swing the weights and let momentum take over.

Breathe. No matter how hard you're working, don't hold your breath! Instead, exhale during the hardest part of the move to push your way through.

Keep your abs active. Even if you're working your biceps, keep your abdominal muscles pulled in and taut. Think of drawing your belly button toward your spine. This not only helps you burn more calories (because you're using more muscles) but also helps you maintain proper form and protects your back as you lift and lower the weights.

you as fun and interesting. Use the log on page 136 to keep track of what you've done each day.

By building shapely, metabolism-revving lean muscle tissue and moving your body with healthy cardiovascular activity, you'll turn your body into a strong, balanced, fat-sizzling machine! And you can lose 30 percent more weight using the *Prevention*'s Shortcuts strategy than you would by following a traditional exercise program. In one study of 56 overweight women, researchers asked half the group to exercise 40 minutes a day all in one shot, while the other half performed four 10-minute bouts. In the end, the short-bout exercisers stuck to the program better (exercising 87 versus 69 days during the study), exercised longer (almost 4 hours a week versus 3), and lost more weight (19½ pounds versus 14 pounds) than those who were stuck with long bouts.

WORKOUT A

For each exercise, do two sets of 12 to 15 repetitions. You can either do both sets of a single exercise consecutively or do one set of every exercise and then repeat.

Squat/Overhead Press

Double-Arm Row

Curtsy Lunge

Pushup

Triceps Overhead Press

Pilates Crunch

SQUAT/OVERHEAD PRESS

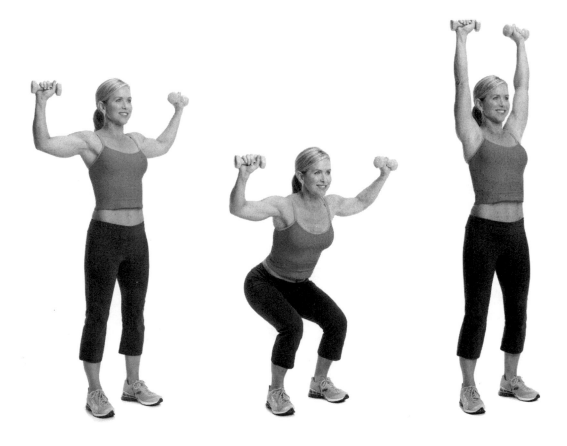

Stand tall with your feet hip-width apart, holding weights in both hands. Begin with your arms bent in the goalpost position: at 90-degree angles out to the sides, with straight wrists and tight abs.

Bend your knees to lower your body into a squat position, going as low as you can but no farther than knees bent to 90 degrees. Pretend you are sitting back into a chair—stick out your buns, keep your chest lifted and spine long, and keep your knees above your ankles.

Push through your heels and squeeze your buns to rise back up. As you reach a standing position, immediately extend your arms to press the weights overhead. Lower them back to the goalpost position.

DOUBLE-ARM ROW

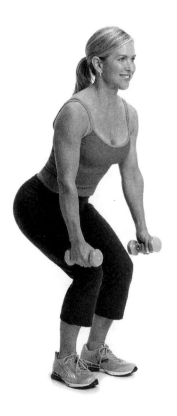 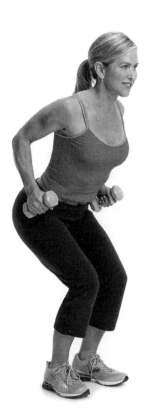

Standing with your feet hip- to shoulder-width apart, knees slightly bent, hold a weight in each hand. Leaning slightly forward from the hips, squat down toward an imaginary chair, keeping your back flat and abs tight. Allow your arms to hang down toward the floor, palms facing in.

Pull your elbows back like you're rowing a boat, and squeeze your shoulder blades together to lift the weights to either side of your ribs. Lower back to the starting position.

CURTSY LUNGE

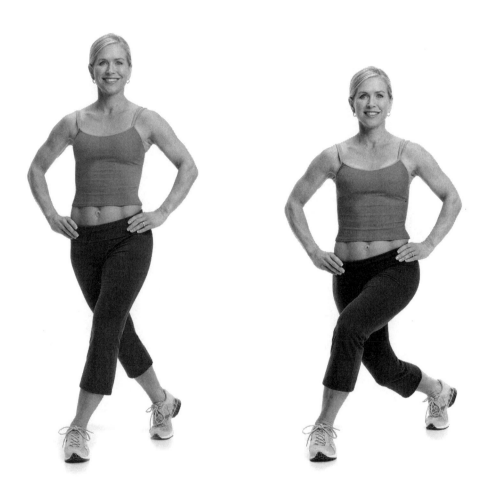

Stand with your feet hip-width apart, hands on your hips. With your right leg, take a giant step back and to the left so that if you were standing on a clock facing 12, your right foot would end up at the 8 o'clock position.

Keeping your back straight and your head up, bend your knees to lower your hips toward the floor until your left thigh is parallel to the ground. Press into your left leg to rise back to the starting position. Complete a full set, then switch sides.

PUSHUP

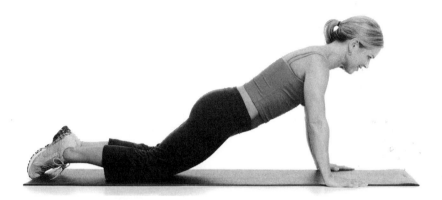

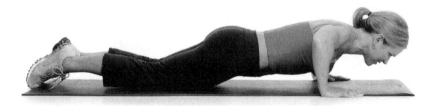

Stretch out on the mat, facedown, in plank position with your arms straight and your hands flat on the floor, a little farther than shoulder-width apart. If you are a beginner, start with your knees on the floor.

Keeping your core tight and level, bend your elbows to 90 degrees to lower your body, keeping your abs tight. Don't sag in the middle. Push back up to the starting position.

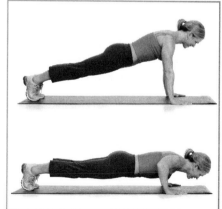

If you are more advanced, rest your toes on the floor, rather than your knees. This takes more core body strength.

TRICEPS OVERHEAD PRESS

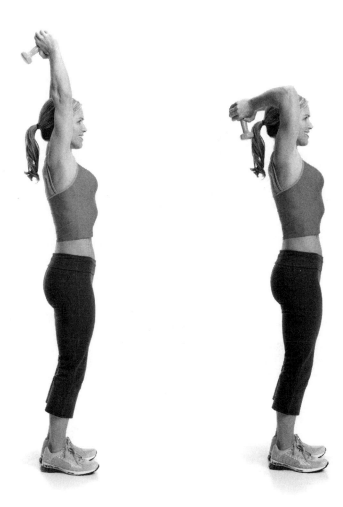

Stand with your feet hip-width apart (or sit in a chair). Clasp one weight with both hands. Extend your arms straight overhead, elbows close to your ears.

Bend your elbows to slowly lower the weight behind you. Keep your elbows close to your ears. Contract your triceps and straighten your elbows to return to the starting position.

PILATES CRUNCH

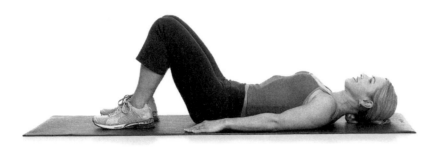

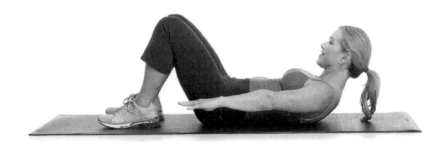

Lie faceup on the floor with your knees bent, your feet hip-width apart and flat on the ground, and your arms at your sides, palms on the floor.

Visualize sliding your rib cage to your pelvis as you pull your navel toward your spine, contract your abs, and sequentially roll your head, shoulders, and upper back off the floor. As you perform the move, lengthen through the back of your neck and tuck your chin slightly toward your chest, while keeping your arms parallel to the floor. Lower back to the starting position. This is the difference between mindlessly crunching and really pulling in and activating your deep transversus abdominis muscles to make your core muscles work.

WORKOUT B

For each exercise, do two sets of 12 to 15 repetitions. You can either do both sets of a single exercise consecutively or do one set of every exercise and then repeat.

Plié

Lateral Raise

Reverse Fly

Stationary Lunge/Hammer Curl

Chest Fly

Half Roll-Back

PLIÉ

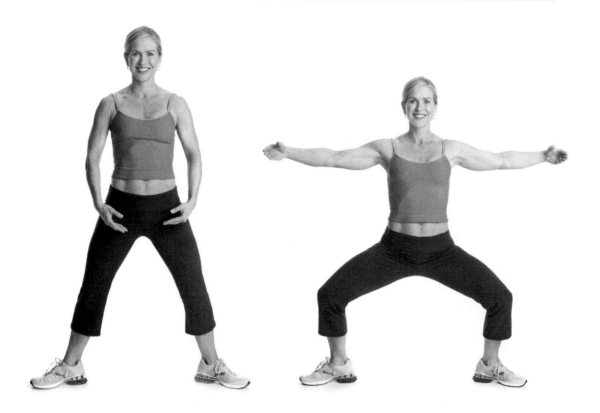

Stand with your feet farther than shoulder-width apart, toes pointing out.

Raise your arms straight out to the sides, palms facing forward. Keeping your back straight, extend your knees over your toes and tuck your tailbone underneath you as if you were sliding down an imaginary wall. Then press into your feet and squeeze your buns to rise back to the starting position.

For a more advanced exercise, deepen your range of motion by trying to get your thighs parallel to the floor.

LATERAL RAISE

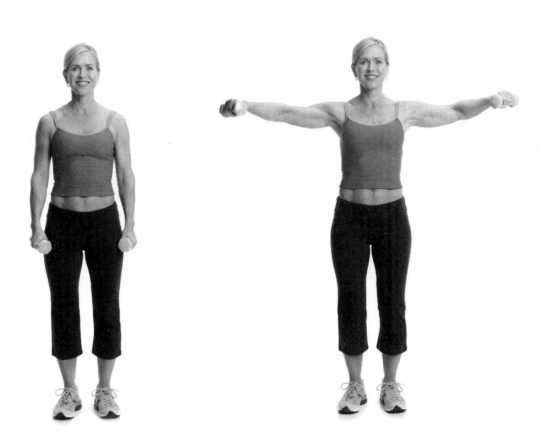

Standing with your feet hip-width apart, hold weights at your sides, palms facing each other.

Keeping your elbows slightly bent, raise your arms straight out to the sides until they are parallel to the floor. Do not raise your arms above shoulder level. Keep your shoulders relaxed—don't shrug! Lower back to the starting position.

REVERSE FLY

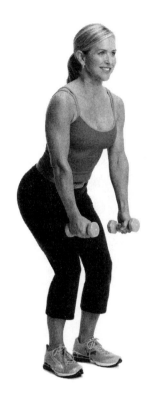 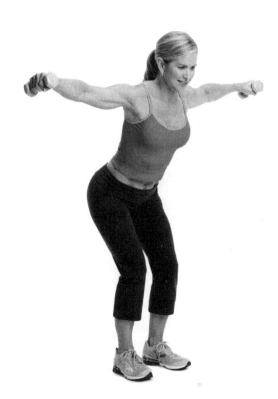

Standing with your feet hip- to shoulder-width apart, knees slightly bent, hold a weight in each hand. Lean slightly forward from the hips, keeping your back flat and abs tight. Allow your arms to hang toward the floor, palms facing each other.

Squeeze your shoulder blades together as you lift the weights, extending your arms out to the sides like airplane wings. Make sure to relax your neck. Don't squeeze or scrunch your shoulders. Lower back to the starting position.

STATIONARY LUNGE/HAMMER CURL

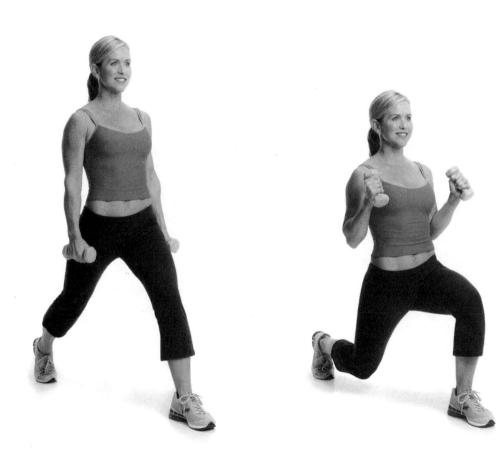

Stand in a split stance: front foot flat on the floor, back heel raised. Hold a weight in each hand, with your palms facing in toward your thighs.

Bend your elbows to curl the weights to your shoulders as you simultaneously bend both knees and lower into a lunge, keeping your front knee directly above the ankle and your back knee pointing down at the floor. Keep your abs tight, chest lifted, and spine long. Lower your body only as far as is comfortable. Don't bend your knees more than 90 degrees. Squeeze through your buns to raise yourself back up to the starting position. Finish a set, then switch legs.

CHEST FLY

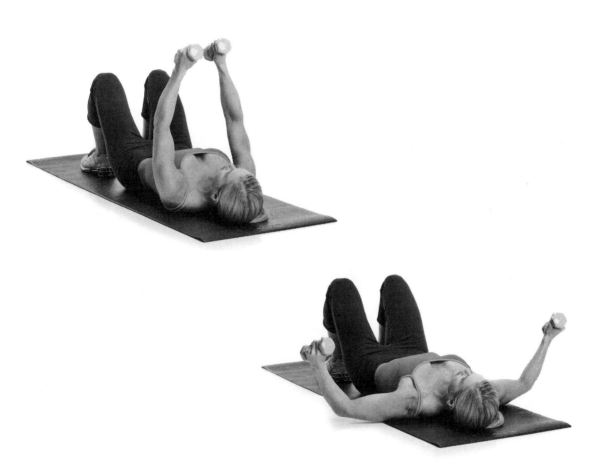

Lie faceup on the floor with your legs bent and your feet flat. Hold weights up over your chest with your arms extended, elbows slightly bent, and palms facing each other.

Slowly open your arms out to the sides, allowing the weights to fall to about the 10 o'clock and 2 o'clock positions. Then slowly lift your arms back to the starting position. Focus on squeezing through your chest as if you were hugging a large tree.

HALF ROLL-BACK

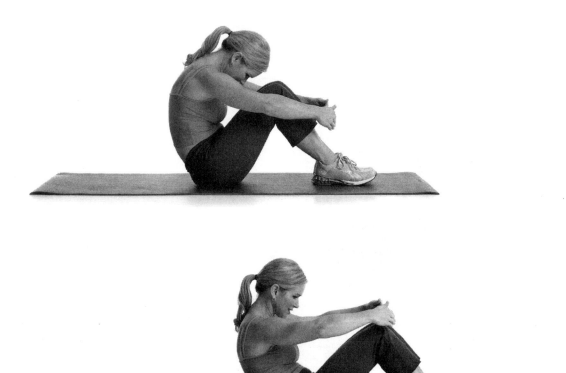

Sit on the floor with your knees bent and your feet and knees separated slightly. Pull your navel toward your spine and curl your spine forward so your torso is bent over your legs in a C shape. Reach your arms forward, with your shoulders relaxed.

Exhale and, maintaining a C shape with your spine, roll halfway back by tucking your tailbone and lowering vertebrae by vertebrae. Inhale and pull your abs even closer toward your spine. Then exhale and contract your abs to return to the starting position. Maintain a rounded spine throughout the movement.

WORKOUT C

For each exercise, do two sets of 12 to 15 repetitions. You can either do both sets of a single exercise consecutively or do one set of every exercise and then repeat.

Simple Squat

Overhead Shoulder Press

Diagonal Lunge/Cross Lift

Triceps Dip on Chair

Bridge/Chest Press

Full-Body Roll-Up

SIMPLE SQUAT

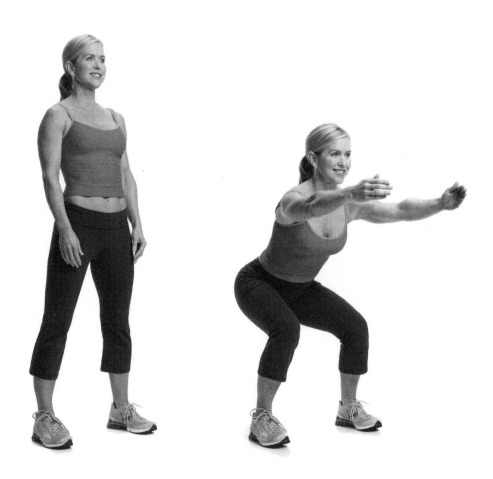

Stand with your feet hip-width apart, toes facing forward, abs tight, and arms at your sides.

Bend your knees to lower your body into a squat position, going as low as you can but no farther than knees bent to 90 degrees. Pretend you are sitting back into a chair—stick out your buns, keep your chest lifted and spine long, and extend your arms out in front of you—and keep your knees above your ankles. Push through your heels and squeeze your buns to rise back to the starting position.

OVERHEAD SHOULDER PRESS

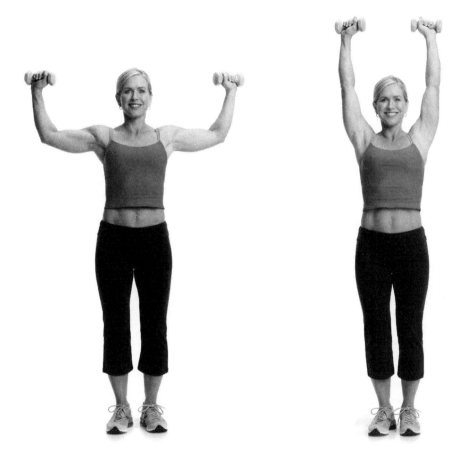

Stand tall with your feet shoulder-width apart, holding weights in both hands. Begin with your arms bent in the goalpost position: at 90-degree angles out to the sides, with straight wrists and tight abs.

Lift your arms overhead until they are straight. Lower back to the starting position.

DIAGONAL LUNGE/CROSS LIFT

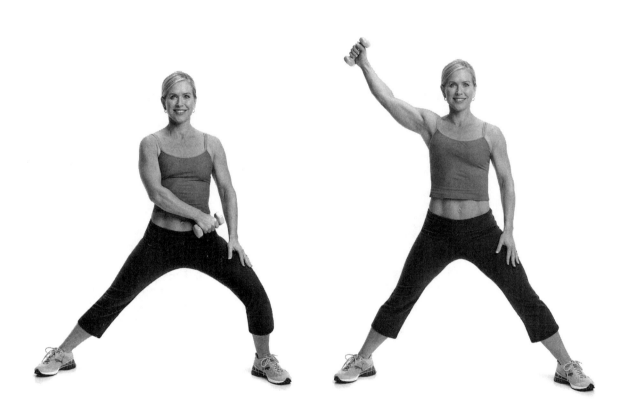

Stand with your legs wide apart in a straddle stance, toes pointed out. Bend your left knee into a 45-degree lunge. Place your left hand on your left thigh. Hold a weight in your right hand and extend your right arm across your body, placing the weight at your left hip, palm facing you.

Press into your left foot and straighten your left leg while simultaneously swinging your right arm across your body and up so it forms a diagonal line with your left leg (as if you were drawing a sword from a scabbard). Return to the starting position. Complete a set, then switch sides.

TRICEPS DIP ON CHAIR

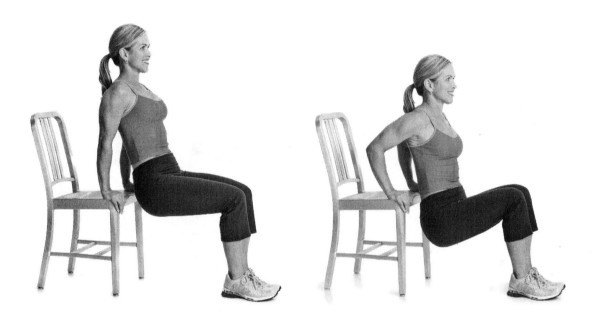

Sit on the edge of a chair, grasping the seat with a hand at either side of your hips. Slide your buns off the seat while walking your feet forward.

Bend your elbows straight back, lowering your hips toward the floor until your elbows are in line with your shoulders. Press back up to the starting position.

Advanced exercisers can straighten one or both legs.

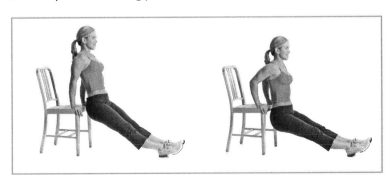

BRIDGE/CHEST PRESS

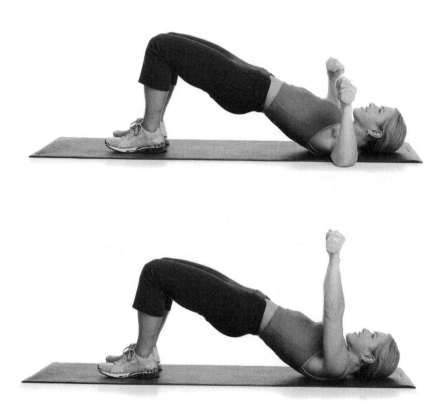

Holding a weight in each hand, lie back on the floor with your knees bent, feet flat on the floor. Hold your forearms perpendicular to the floor and position the weights at either side of your chest, ends facing one another. Keeping your hips square to the ceiling and your navel pulled toward your spine, press into your heels, squeeze your buns, and lift your hips toward the ceiling so your body forms a straight line from your knees to your shoulders.

Extend your arms to press the weights straight up. Pause, then return to the starting position.

FULL-BODY ROLL-UP

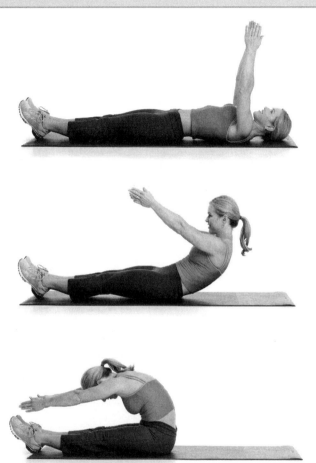

Lie faceup on the floor with your arms relaxed and extended straight up. Pull your navel toward your spine to engage your abdominal muscles as you inhale and stretch your arms upward.

Exhale, lengthen the back of your neck, tuck your chin toward your chest, and, keeping your navel pulled toward your spine, curl forward with your arms extending in front of you. Visualize leading with the top of your head to create a C curve, curling forward until you are reaching for your toes. Inhale as you stay rounded.

Begin reversing direction, uncurling your body. Exhale as you continue to "drip" your spine back to the floor, one vertebrae at a time, slowly lowering back to the starting position.

BIG WEIGHT LOSS LOG

Make photocopies of this log and use them to keep track of each and every one of the *Prevention*'s Shortcuts you take. Three to 5 days a week, you want to check off at least one Big Weight Loss workout. Check off one of the cardio walking workouts every day, and at least 3 days a week do a second one. Also remember to give yourself extra credit for every 1-Minute Wonder and Lifestyle Shortcut you squeeze in.

	SUN	MON	TUES	WED	THU	FRI	SAT
Big Weight Loss							
Workout A							
Workout B							
Workout C							
Cardio (see Chapter 4)							
Need for Speed							
Fast and Focused							
Strong and Steady							
Pyramid Power							
Rolling Hills							
Conquer the Mountain							
1-Minute Wonder							
Let Your Feet Do the Walking (page 36)							
Tap Your Toes! (page 76)							
Do "Invisible" Exercise (page 99)							
Multitasking Moves (page 149)							
Stealth Leg Slimmers (page 243)							
Sneaky Arm Shapers (page 295)							

	SUN	MON	TUES	WED	THU	FRI	SAT
Armchair Athletics (page 328)							
Lifestyle Shortcut							
Walk This Way (page 77)							
Take It Outside! (page 80)							
Take Action! (page 144)							
Just Say No (page 178)							
Use Flower Power (page 179)							
Think Positive! (page 180)							
Get Sleep! (page 190)							
Drink Up! (page 191)							
Laugh It Up . . . and Off (page 297)							
Hit the Pound (page 299)							
Hoop It Up (page 329)							
Step Up to the Plate (page 358)							
Live for the Future (page 360)							

Notes (goals, feelings, etc.): _____

_____

_____

_____

_____

_____

_____

_____

_____

REFRESH YOUR MEMORY

Still not finding time to fit in the exercise for big weight loss? Go back to Chapter 2 and reread some of the answers you gave in the quizzes to identify your barriers (and, of course, the answers to overcoming them). Remember, you can do these exercises while you watch TV. You can do them while your baby naps. You *can* do it. Just remind yourself of all those reasons you really want it.

I'm a big believer in daily affirmations and mantras. Seventy percent of the time we talk to ourselves, we're saying something negative. I tell my aerobics classes 20 times an hour, "You guys are awesome!" It's like subliminal messaging. They hear it as they are sweating and moving, and it sinks into their subconscious! Take that extra step and jot down why you're working out and how you're going to make it happen. Use a positive "I want . . . So I will . . . " format. For instance:

10-SECOND WISDOM

"There's an athlete in us all. Let her out to play!"

I want . . .

To ride a bike without feeling out of breath.

So I will . . .

Do a 10-minute cardio interval workout at lunch, and do 10 minutes of strength training after dinner tonight.

I want . . .

To feel proud when I walk into my class reunion this summer.

So I will . . .

Lose weight by doing three *Prevention*'s Shortcuts workouts and implementing Clean-Eating Shortcuts every day for 8 weeks—the amount of time it takes to make a behavior a habit.

Make your "I want . . . So I will . . . " statements as specific and personal as possible for the best results.

Prevention's Shortcuts Success Story

"I HAVE LOST 230 POUNDS."

You read that right. When I started working out, my weight was 396 pounds and I was a size 28. I had tried every diet known to man, but I never exercised and always gained the weight back. As a single mother of two boys, ages 7 and 10, I became afraid that I was on a slow path to death and was going to leave them alone in the world. I woke up one day and decided to make a lifestyle change.

The hardest part was getting started. Now I can't imagine stopping. I move whenever possible. When I'm watching TV, I get up and do something during every commercial. Even if I have to stay up 15 minutes later or get up 30 minutes earlier, I make sure to work out every day. I make exercising as much a part of my life as I do with brushing my teeth or doing laundry, and I have more energy through my day as a result. I love knowing I will live longer for my boys, and being able to climb stairs without being winded, and being able to keep up with my boys as we ride bikes, play football, or play in the park. The best part is that *anyone* can do these workouts. You don't have to be a size 2 or weigh 115 pounds. Any age, fitness level, or size can do them. No excuses.

Amy, 32

FOLLOW THE FOOD RULES

Exercise takes care of burning calories and excess stored fat. But when you want to lose lots of weight, that's only half the equation. You must, must, must pay close attention to the calories that are coming in. Most women who are eager to lose weight try to starve themselves thin (and they inevitably regain the weight). I want you to eat!

You're going to need plenty of fuel for your *Prevention's* Shortcuts workouts. Only now we'll make sure the food you eat is "clean" (that's as close to its real form in nature).

Though I do meet some women who have trouble with binge eating (usually those who starve themselves most of the day, then gorge at night because they're so hungry and feel deprived), most of my clients take in excess calories through mindless munching: a cookie or two from the office pantry here; a pack of M&M'S from the vending machine there. Following the Clean-Eating Shortcuts throughout the book will curb this type of toxic grazing by reminding you to be more aware of every morsel you put in your mouth. Even better: Once you start eating clean, whole foods, you'll feel so much better, you won't be nearly as tempted by refined salty or sugary snack foods filled with artificial flavors and colors. This is a *very* important step to grasp for big weight loss. Remember, it all boils down to calories, and you have to lose 3,500 through diet and exercise to lose a pound. It sounds like a big number, but if you just cut 250 calories a day by controlling your portions and skipping one sugary snack or swapping plain grilled chicken for buffalo wings, then burn 250 a day through your *Prevention's* Shortcuts workouts (which you'll do automatically), you can lose 52 pounds in a year while barely even thinking about it!

10-SECOND WISDOM

"It takes a few days for the body to react to its newfound energy. But you'll be surprised by how great you feel—even if you didn't know you weren't feeling good before! I had a client say after kicking her fast-food addiction and eating healthier, 'I didn't know I felt so bad until I starting seeing how good I could really feel!'"

Whatever you do, don't deprive yourself. If you feel like you're missing out on all the tastes you love, you'll be cruising the dessert aisle within a week. Instead, figure out how to get the flavors and food satisfaction you want in healthier ways. For instance, if you have a sweet tooth, try one of my favorite smoothie drinks: In a blender, combine 1 cup of 1% milk, ½ cup of low-fat vanilla yogurt, ½ cup of frozen berries, half a banana, and 2 tablespoons of flaxseed. It'll give you the smooth, sweet satisfaction of ice cream without all the calories. One of my clients who loves rich salad dressings found that slicing avocados on her lunch salad gives her the creaminess she craves without the unhealthy fat and sugar calories. And, of course, don't forget to let yourself have the real thing, whether it's cheesecake or a cheesesteak, three or four times a month. Life is too short to completely forgo your favorite foods.

STAY OFF THE SCALE

Generally speaking, the bathroom scale can be a good way to measure progress and keep you on the path to your weight loss goals. But it can also be a giant source of frustration for women starting the *Prevention's* Shortcuts program—not because you're not getting results (you most definitely will) but because they're not accurately reflected in numbers on the scale.

CLEAN-EATING SHORTCUT
HAVE IT YOUR WAY

On any given day, half of all Americans will eat out at a restaurant. Dining out has gone from a once-in-a-while treat to an essential part of our eating habits. That means we can't treat every restaurant experience as an indulgence, dipping slice after slice of sourdough into the olive oil pool, choosing rich entrées, and ordering dessert. But let's face it, once we walk through the restaurant doors, many of us mindlessly slip into that behavior. It's almost automatic. The trick is to "order" your food in your mind before you get there.

I know some women who actually look up the menu online and choose what they want in their heads before they arrive, so they have the luxury of deciding on the healthiest selections before they get a whiff of the blue cheese–smothered steak. But you certainly don't have to go to that extreme! Whether it's an Italian bistro or a Mexican joint, you can bet on standard dishes—like pasta with marinara or grilled chicken fajitas—being available. Decide what types of healthy dishes you will look for before you go, choosing clear broths over cream sauces, grilled or broiled dishes over fried, and so on. Also determine ahead of time that you will eat just three nachos or a half slice of bread. Then, once you get to the restaurant, all your choices are already made, so you're more likely to stick to them.

Remember, every bite counts. Don't leave them up to chance. Even if you can't see the menu online, you can still order what you want, how you want it, at most places. I've learned to always ask for my entrée the way I want it—grilled, sauce on the side, extra veggies, no potatoes, you name it. My husband used to be embarrassed; now he wants me to order for him, too!

Let me explain. If you've been sedentary for a long time, or if you've never really done strength training before, your body composition is likely disproportionately skewed toward fat. I probably don't have to tell you that fat tissue takes up a lot of space, but what you may not know is that, inch for inch, it weighs considerably less than dense, svelte muscle tissue. That's why you can have one 140-pound woman who wears a size 6 and another who wears a size 10 or larger, even though they weigh the same. So as you are doing your *Prevention*'s Shortcuts workouts and losing fat and building muscle, you may find that the numbers on the scale aren't dropping as quickly as your waistline is shrinking.

Better ways to measure your progress include watching how your clothes fit or taking circumference measurements. By using a tape measure to measure your waist, hips, thighs, and upper arms, you can see the results that matter—you're losing excess inches. Also, don't forget your mirror. Looking at your reflection and seeing healthy skin, a trimmer silhouette, and shapely muscles starting to peek through is the greatest measurement of success of all.

DRESS FOR SUCCESS

I'm not a fashion expert, but I do know that clothes reflect the way a woman feels about herself. I want you to feel good about yourself, and I can tell you that if you're wearing a giant baggy T-shirt, it's probably not doing the trick. Too many women who are unhappy with their weight try to hide themselves in big, baggy clothes, which often have the opposite effect.

You know all those impressive before-and-after pictures you see in women's magazines? While many of them *have* lost impressive amounts of weight, others haven't lost more than 5 or 10 pounds, yet they look like they've lost 20. Why is that? It's not trick photography or Photoshop. It's the clothes. When the stylist comes in to prep them for the after pictures, she is careful to dress them in stylish, figure-flattering activewear, instead of the big, baggy shirts and slacks the women usually show up in for the before shots. Sharp dressing is the quickest way I know to look 10 pounds slimmer. If you haven't already, check out the advice on page 38 to find places to stock up on affordable, feel-good-look-great clothes for women of all sizes. I guarantee that if you slip into just one or two pretty, more formfitting outfits, people will start asking you if you lost weight before you shed an ounce.

Here's the most important part. As you lose weight, ceremoniously ditch some of

Prevention's Shortcuts Success Story

"IT ALL ADDS UP!"

I made a commitment to work out at 5:30 a.m. most days. If I can't make it in the morning, I try to squeeze it in during the evening. If neither of those works, I make sure I get out and move my body some other way during the day, whether it be a walk or a bike ride. I've learned that every bit of activity adds up, so it's important to find a way to move. So far, I've lost 70 pounds. Before I lost the weight, I was wearing a size 20. Now I'm in a 10. I haven't weighed this little in over 16 years. I've had my setbacks along the way, but I keep an old picture of myself before I lost the weight on the nightstand by my bed. That picture reminds me how hard I have worked and how far I've come.

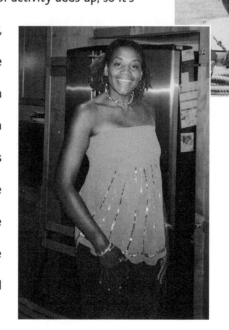

Toya, 42

your too-big clothes and replace them with a few new pieces. This doesn't have to be a huge, expensive wardrobe makeover. But you need to acknowledge in a meaningful way that the new you is here to stay. By squirreling away all those oversize clothes, you send a message to your subconscious that this change is temporary. With the *Prevention*'s Shortcuts system, it's here to stay!

LIFESTYLE SHORTCUT
TAKE ACTION!

Psychologists tell us we go through five distinct stages whenever we make a major change in our livres, whether it's quitting smoking or launching healthy lifestyle changes like eating well and exercising. The first is precontemplation, in which you haven't even thought about changing yet. You may not even think there's a problem. Next is contemplation, where you are seriously thinking about change but haven't done anything about it. Preparation, the third stage, is when you start laying the groundwork to make a change. The act of buying this book is preparation. Next comes action. Unless you want to get stuck in preparation—or worse, forget this book in a dusty corner and slip back to contemplation—you need to move today!

The final stage is maintenance. Once you've made your changes and gotten your results, you continue your healthy new habits to maintain your positive gains. Everyone hits maintenance at a different rate. Some women may hit it in 2 months. Others may take a year or longer. It doesn't matter how long it takes, just that you get there.

CHAPTER 6

Blast Through a Plateau

(And Finally Shed Those Last 10 Pounds!)

It's not your imagination. It really *does* get harder to lose weight as you get older. And those annoying 10 or 12 pounds you used to be able to drop with a few weeks of "good behavior" seem to stick around your hips, belly, and thighs no matter what you do.

Making matters worse, our lives get crazier as we get older. Between aging parents and demanding kids, hectic jobs and community responsibilities, there's less time left just for us. That's why I wrote *Prevention*'s Shortcuts just for you. Instead of waiting for life to calm down (which it won't), you can seize every moment right now to get your old body back—and to do it faster than you would with conventional 30- to 40-minute workouts.

KEEP YOUR EYE ON THE PRIZE

I'll be totally honest: Losing those last 10 pounds will not happen overnight. Whereas those initial pounds seem to come flying off when you have a lot to lose, the closer you get to your goal weight, the slower progress seems to become. For one, your body is inclined to hang on to those reserves "just in case," so you're fighting Mother Nature. But also, at this point, you're just tweaking an already pretty healthy lifestyle,

Prevention's Shortcuts Success Story
"I'M MAKING A 10-MINUTE COMEBACK!"

I went from a size 12 to a size 10 in just 4 weeks. . . . After seeing a difference in my body's appearance and feeling better in just 4 weeks of these tiny changes, I'm now confident that, yes, I can do more and keep going. . . . My clothes are fitting better, and my wardrobe has expanded since I can now fit back into things that were too tight.

For me, the most electrifying aspect of Chris's workouts is that they build confidence and drive and make it easier to change my mind-set and attitude about fitness and wellness. Other workouts have an intimidation factor because the movements look jarring and diffi-cult . . . and the trainers who do them look like they'd get angry if I missed a workout. Chris is not here to "manage" our fitness lives—she is a fitness leader, and leaders engage people to make good decisions, take ownership of their bodies and healthful lifestyle, and, above all, make us feel good about each and every movement we make.

Each 10-minute segment of movement has helped me to rebuild my confidence and interest in working out, staying healthy, and challenging my body to be the best it can.

Kate, 33

so the weight loss is less dramatic. Yes, it can be frustrating. But if you throw in the towel, it won't happen at all!

To keep from getting discouraged, you need to be as positive as possible. When jotting your progress in the workout log on page 174, make note of everything that made you feel good about that workout. Were you proud of yourself for getting up 10 minutes early? Write it down. Did you feel more energetic during a big day at work?

Do you find yourself sleeping more soundly at night? Exercise and eating right bestow so many great things on our lives, it's important to appreciate *all* of the benefits along the path to our weight loss goals.

Finally, give yourself a break now and then, and remember what's important in life. So what if the kitchen stays dirty for a night? Don't stress the mess. Let it go—especially if it means you get the chance to get in a good workout. Resist the urge to compare yourself to others. So many women look next door and see a perfect house with a totally chic woman going off to her high-powered job, and they feel deflated because they don't "measure up." The green-eyed monster of envy and jealousy will eat away your energy and, in many cases, send you to the fridge for consolation. Don't let it take hold of you. Trust me, every woman has her issues. We all make compromises somewhere. Keep your eyes on your goals and what's good in your life.

The secret to losing those last stubborn pounds is to fire up your metabolism by getting your heart rate up higher than you usually do, throwing your muscles and cardiovascular system a surprise curveball to bump your fitness to the next level. I'm a creature of change—I can't stand to do the same form of exercise day after day, and I think that's a big part of the reason I manage to keep my weight steady year after year. That's why in this chapter, in between the strengthening exercises, I've built in Cardio Quick Takes exercises from Chapter 4. The high-energy cardio moves not only maximize calorie burning but also add variety to keep your body guessing and your mind from getting bored.

Additionally, the strengthening exercises themselves are designed to keep your heart rate high because they work many muscles at once. By blending, for instance, your biceps curls with your lunges, you work more of your muscles in a shorter period of time. That means faster toning and a higher calorie burn per exercise session. What's more, these moves improve your balance, coordination, and core strength, because your body needs to fire up all those supporting muscles in your abs and back to stabilize your torso while you lift with your arms and legs. This is a multitasker's dream—getting two, three, maybe four or five muscles toned in one move!

PEAKS, PLATEAUS, AND PROGRESS

To appreciate the benefit of combination moves, it helps to understand a little of the science behind strength training. When you first pick up hand weights and start doing presses and curls, your brain gets the message that your muscles are in for some serious work and could use a little help. So it starts forging new neuromuscular connections, literally pathways from your central nervous system to your muscles, recruiting new muscle fibers to help get the job done. That's when you see some of your greatest—and fastest—fitness gains. As you recruit and strengthen more muscle fibers, you lose fat and gain shapely muscle tone. You also get stronger. Slamming a tennis serve feels easier, as does schlepping an overflowing basket of laundry down one or two flights of stairs.

10-SECOND WISDOM

"Most people are imprisoned by inertia. If you force yourself to start moving, momentum—and maybe even motivation—is likely to follow."

Eventually, however, those strength gains slow to a halt. As those same squats and presses become easier, your muscles use fewer fibers to get the job done. That's when you need to pick up some heavier weights and give your muscles a fresh challenge. But let's face it, there's only so much weight a woman can lift (you and I won't be pressing 80-pounders anytime soon). Unless you do something to give your muscles a little kick in the pants, you'll hit a plateau.

Plateaus are those stubborn sticking points where, seemingly out of nowhere, your progress comes to a screeching halt and those jeans you seemed so close to squeezing into still won't zip. We all hit those walls. The combination moves in this chapter are my secret weapon for blasting through those walls and losing those last 10 to 12 pounds.

By doing these moves that simultaneously target the large muscles in your glutes, legs, back, and chest, you not only activate those major muscle groups but also get the supporting muscles in your core buzzing as they work to stabilize your torso as you move your limbs. Because your muscles are working in new ways, you'll forge new neuromuscular connections and strengthen new fibers. Working your upper and lower body together also raises your heart rate so you'll get a mini cardio kick. In the end, you'll shake up all those slumbering muscles and put your results back on fast-forward.

Finally, I love these moves because they're so functional. Rarely in life are you standing perfectly still while using just your biceps to lift something from your legs to your shoulders. Instead, you're squatting down on one leg to grab a bag of groceries with one hand while you try to open the car door with the other. Life involves your arms, legs, back, and chest working together in harmony. These multijoint moves will help you be strong for life.

Thanks to this unique plateau-busting combination of exercises and the Clean-Eating Shortcuts you learned in Chapter 3, you can expect to lose up to 2 pounds per week, so you can finally shed those last 10 pounds in a little more than a month. Do one workout from this chapter 3 to 5 days a week. If you feel highly motivated or have extra time, you can do more than one workout in a day, but that's not necessary. I've provided three different Plateau Buster workouts—A, B, and C—and you can choose whichever one(s) you like, though I recommend mixing them up rather than doing the same one every time. Also do plenty of cardio—at least one of the Chapter 4 workouts every day, plus a second one of those workouts 3 to 5 days a week. And whenever possible, try a Lifestyle Shortcut, a 1-Minute Wonder, or any of the *Prevention*'s Shortcuts workouts from any other chapters in the book that strike you as fun and interesting. Use the log on page 174 to keep track of what you've done each day.

1-MINUTE WONDER
MULTITASKING MOVES

Shortcut slots are everywhere! Here are some of my favorite ways to include little shots of strength training in my everyday routine, above and beyond my regular *Prevention*'s Shortcuts workouts.

Squeeze in squats. Do squats during commercials, tapping your butt on the edge of a chair with each rep. Squat while chatting on the phone. Your legs literally carry you through life. The stronger and more resilient they are, the better!

Shop and curl. As you shop, do biceps curls. Lift your packages or handbag several times in each arm while perusing the shelves for the right brand to buy.

Tune in to pushups. When you're lying on the floor watching TV, roll over during commercials and do 10 quick pushups.

Step up to calf raises. Holding on to a banister for balance, place the ball of one foot on the edge of a step and raise the other foot slightly so it's off the step. Press your heel downward and upward several times, then repeat with your other leg.

Work in dips. Do triceps dips off your chair at work for a 30-second exercise break.

Perform comforter crunches. Draw your knees to your chest 25 to 50 times before you get out of bed in the morning.

WORKOUT A

Do 12 to 15 repetitions of each of the strength exercises, and do each Cardio Quick Takes exercise for 1 minute. Then repeat the whole workout.

Knee Lift/Single-Arm Row

Power Jab Drill

Squat/Overhead Press

Ski Hop

Curtsy Lunge/Biceps Curl

Basketball Jump Shot

Straight-Leg Reverse Curl

KNEE LIFT/SINGLE-ARM ROW

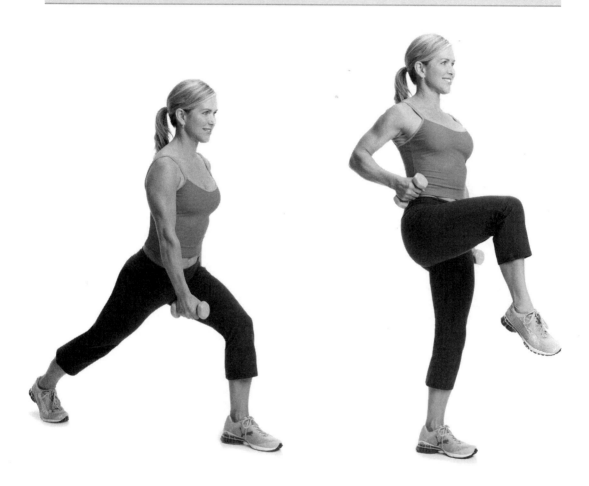

Hold a dumbbell in each hand with your arms at your sides, palms facing in. Take a giant step forward with your left leg.

Lift your right leg up until your thigh is parallel to the floor. At the same time, bend your right elbow to bring the dumbbell up to your rib cage. Return to the starting position. Complete a set on your right side, then switch to your left.

POWER JAB DRILL

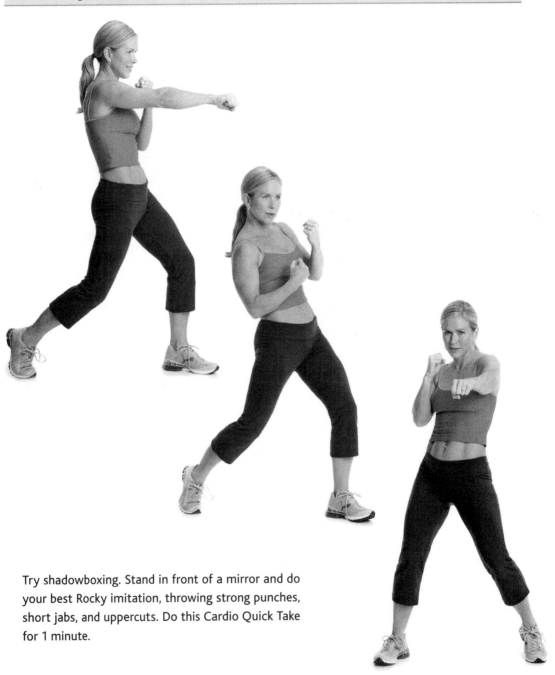

Try shadowboxing. Stand in front of a mirror and do your best Rocky imitation, throwing strong punches, short jabs, and uppercuts. Do this Cardio Quick Take for 1 minute.

SQUAT/OVERHEAD PRESS

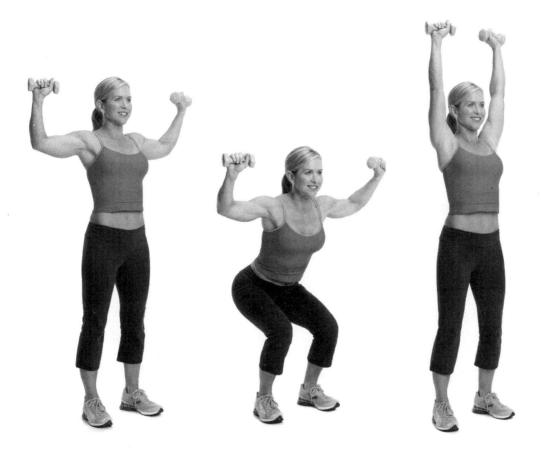

Stand tall with your feet hip-width apart, holding weights in both hands. Begin with your arms bent in the goalpost position: at 90-degree angles out to the sides, with straight wrists and tight abs.

Bend your knees to lower your body into a squat position, going as low as you can but no farther than knees bent to 90 degrees. Pretend you are sitting back into a chair—stick out your buns, keep your chest lifted and spine long, and keep your knees above your ankles.

Push through your heels and squeeze your buns to rise back up. As you reach a standing position, immediately extend your arms to press the weights overhead. Lower them back to the goalpost position.

SKI HOP

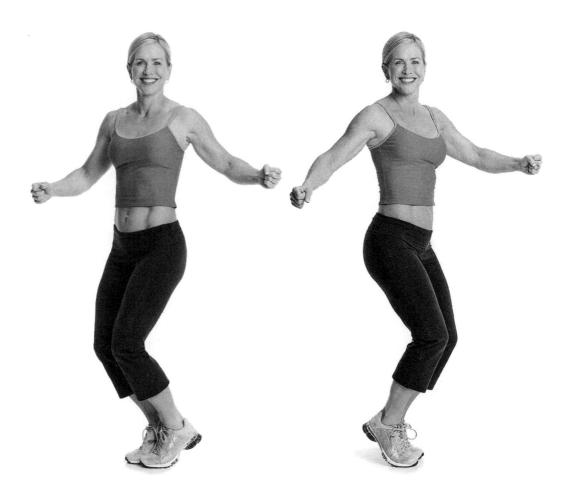

With your feet together, jump from side to side, landing with your knees bent. The wider you jump and the lower you squat into the jump, the harder you'll work. Do this Cardio Quick Take for 1 minute.

CURTSY LUNGE/BICEPS CURL

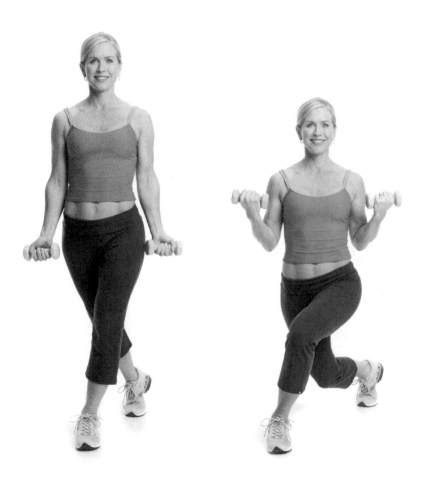

Standing with your feet hip-width apart, hold a weight in each hand, arms down at your sides and palms facing forward. With your right leg, take a giant step back and to the left so that if you were standing on a clock facing 12, your right foot would end up at the 8 o'clock position.

Keeping your back straight and your head up, bend your knees to lower your hips toward the floor until your left thigh is parallel to the floor. At the same time, bend your elbows to curl the weights up to your shoulders. Press into your left leg to rise back to the starting position. Complete a set, then switch sides.

BASKETBALL JUMP SHOT

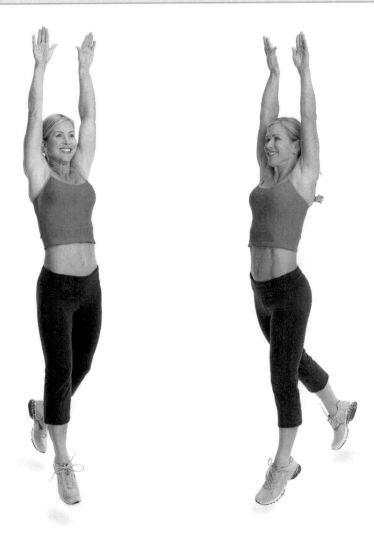

Pretend to shoot some hoops. Step forward on one foot and hop up into the air as if to dunk a basketball. Alternate feet, stepping and hopping. You can step up onto a step to add intensity. Do this Cardio Quick Take for 1 minute.

STRAIGHT-LEG REVERSE CURL

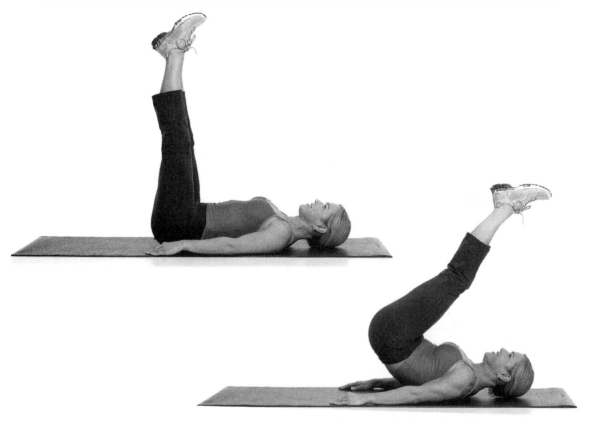

Lie faceup on the floor with your arms at your sides, legs extended into the air at a 90-degree angle to your tailbone on the mat.

Draw your navel toward your spine to scoop your abs and curl your hips off the floor so your feet move slightly over your head. Hold for a moment, then slowly lower back to the starting position.

If your hamstrings are tight, keep your knees slightly bent throughout this exercise.

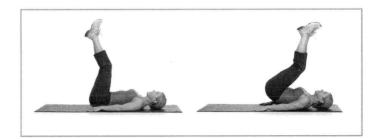

WORKOUT B

Do 12 to 15 repetitions of each of the strength exercises, and do each Cardio Quick Takes exercise for 1 minute. Then repeat the whole workout.

Reverse Lunge/Lateral Raise

Stair Blaster

Deadlift/Double-Arm Row

Squat Hop

Triceps Pressback/Glute Squeeze

Lighting the Torch

Bicycle

REVERSE LUNGE/LATERAL RAISE

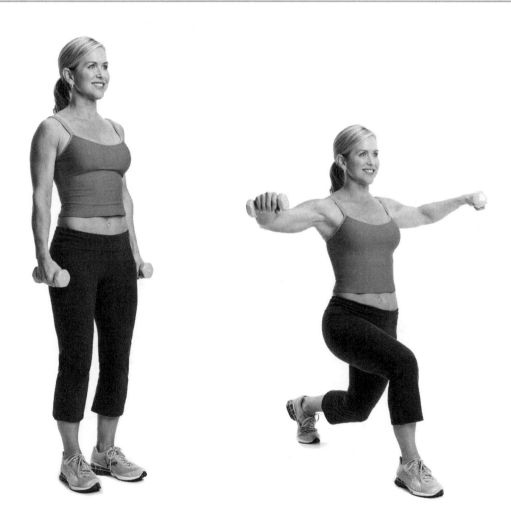

Stand with your feet hip-width apart, holding weights down by your sides, palms facing in.

Take a giant step back with your left leg, then bend your knees to lower your hips toward the floor until your right thigh is parallel to the floor. As you lower, simultaneously lift the weights straight out from your sides until both arms are parallel to the floor. Press back up to the starting position, lowering the weights as you come back to a stand. Complete a set, then switch legs.

STAIR BLASTER

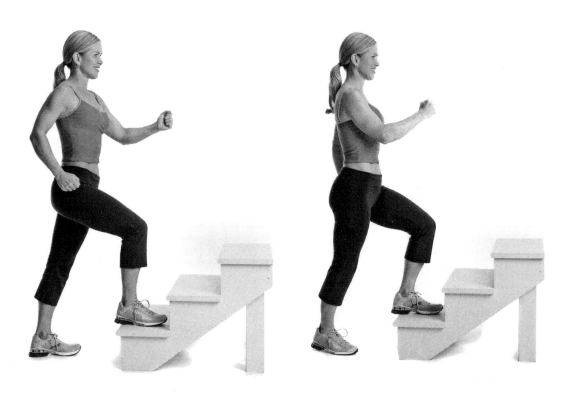

Stand facing a step. Briskly step up with your right and left foot and then down with your right and left foot. Do this Cardio Quick Take for 1 minute.

DEADLIFT/DOUBLE-ARM ROW

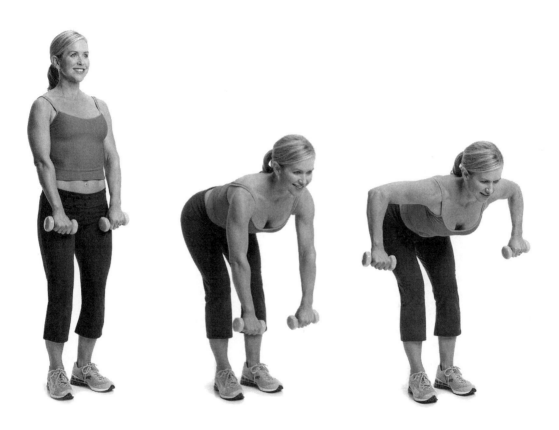

Holding weights down in front of your thighs, palms facing you, stand with your feet hip-width apart and your knees slightly bent.

Keeping your lower back straight, slowly bend at the hips, lowering the weights toward the floor as far as comfortably possible. (Keep the weights close to your body as you lower.)

Once in the down position, pull your elbows back like you're rowing a boat and squeeze your shoulder blades together to lift the weights to either side of your ribs. Lower the weights, then return to the starting position.

SQUAT HOP

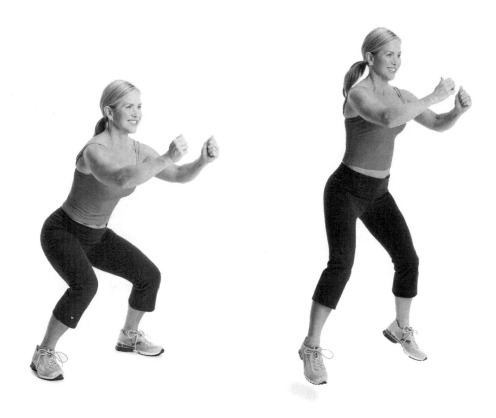

Stand with your feet wide. Lower into a squat and hop forward four times, keeping your feet wide and your legs bent into a squat. Walk back and repeat. Do this Cardio Quick Take for 1 minute.

TRICEPS PRESSBACK/GLUTE SQUEEZE

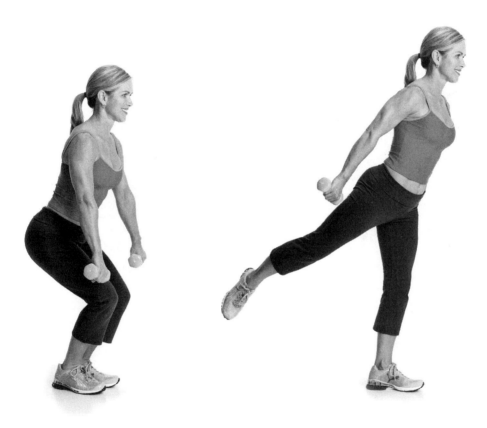

Stand with a weight in each hand, arms extended in front of your thighs, palms facing back. Bend your knees 45 degrees to lower yourself into a partial squat.

Extend your right leg behind you, squeezing your right glute to press your right foot toward the back of the room. At the same time, press your arms straight back, keeping them extended, so your triceps engage. Return to the starting position. On the next rep, extend your left leg.

LIGHTING THE TORCH

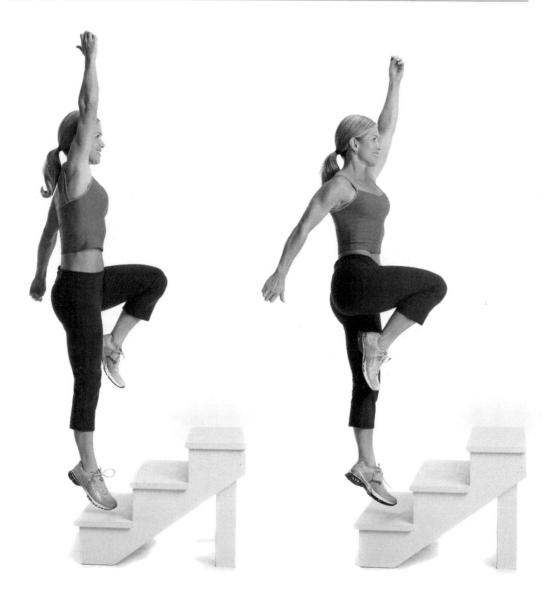

Stand on the floor in front of a staircase, and step onto the bottom step with your right foot while simultaneously lifting your left knee and right arm. Step back down to the floor with your left foot and then your right, then immediately step up with your left foot while raising your right knee and left arm.

BICYCLE

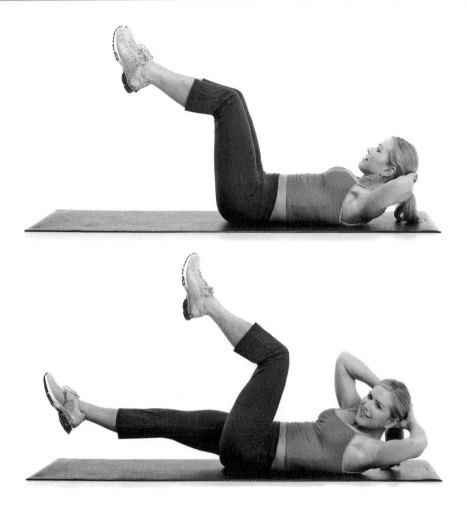

Lie faceup on the floor with your hips and knees bent to about 90-degree angles and your abs tight to protect your lower back. With your hands behind your head, carefully lift your head and shoulders off the floor.

Pull your left knee toward your chest while extending your right leg straight out, parallel to the floor. At the same time, lift and twist your torso to bring your right elbow toward your left knee. Return to the starting position, then repeat on the other side.

WORKOUT C

Do 12 to 15 repetitions of each of the strength exercises, and do each Cardio Quick Takes exercise for 1 minute. Then repeat the whole workout.

Power March

Diagonal Lunge/Cross Lift

Speed Skating

Squat/Overhead Press

Tire Drill

Pushup/Glute-Squeeze Leg Lift

Double-Leg Stretch

POWER MARCH

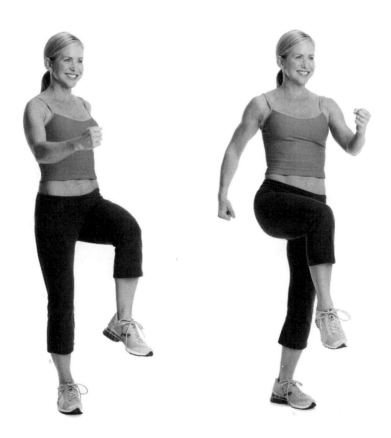

March in place, lifting your knees high as you pump your arms to get your heart rate up. Do this Cardio Quick Take for 1 minute.

DIAGONAL LUNGE/CROSS LIFT

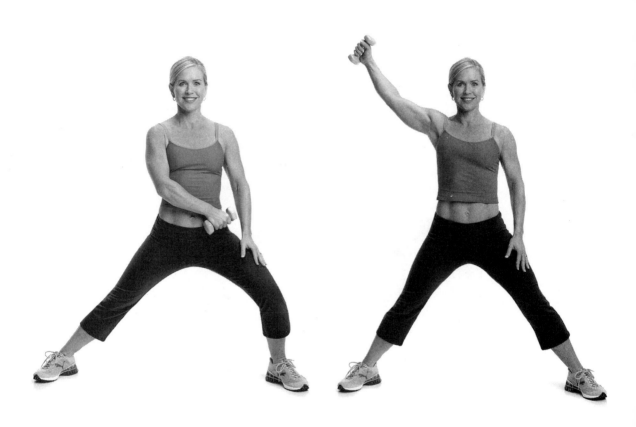

Stand with your legs wide apart in a straddle stance, toes pointed out. Bend your left knee into a 45-degree lunge. Place your left hand on your left thigh. Hold a weight in your right hand and extend your right arm across your body, placing the weight at your left hip, palm facing you.

Press into your left foot and straighten your left leg while simultaneously swinging your right arm across your body and up so it forms a diagonal line with your left leg (as if you were drawing a sword from a scabbard). Return to the starting position. Complete a set, then switch sides.

SPEED SKATING

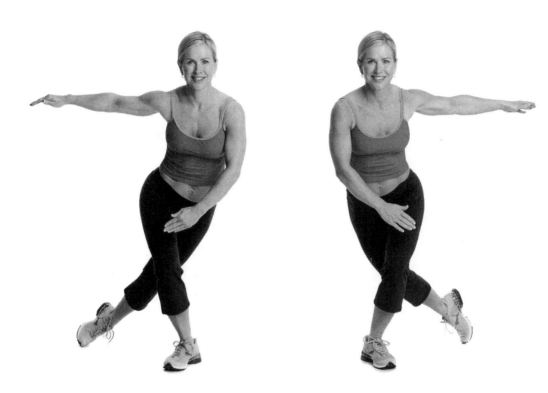

Starting with your feet together, bend your knees and, with your right leg, jump to your right, keeping your body low and landing with a bent right knee. Immediately sweep your left foot behind your right ankle, push off, and jump to your left. Do this Cardio Quick Take for 1 minute.

SQUAT/OVERHEAD PRESS

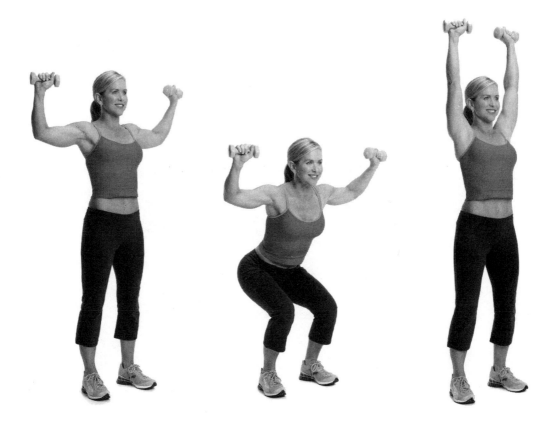

Stand tall with your feet hip-width apart, holding weights in both hands. Begin with your arms bent in the goalpost position: at 90-degree angles out to the sides, with straight wrists and tight abs.

Bend your knees to lower your body into a squat position, going as low as you can but no farther than knees bent to 90 degrees. Pretend you are sitting back into a chair—stick out your buns, keep your chest lifted and spine long, and extend your arms out in front of you—and keep your knees above your ankles.

Push through your heels and squeeze your buns to rise back up. As you reach a standing position, immediately extend your arms to press the weights overhead. Lower them back to the goalpost position.

TIRE DRILL

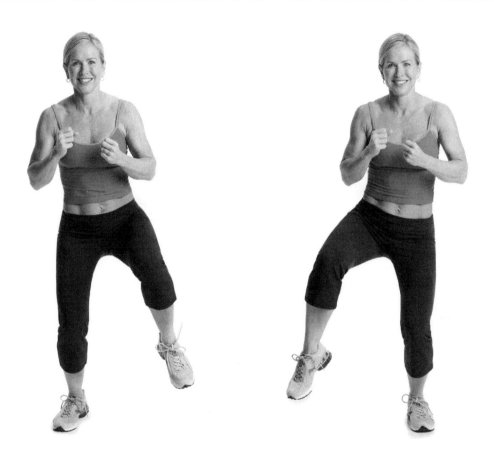

Standing with your feet wide apart and your knees bent about 45 degrees, lift one knee and then the other, taking short quick steps forward as though you were running through tires. Do this Cardio Quick Take for 1 minute.

PUSHUP/GLUTE-SQUEEZE LEG LIFT

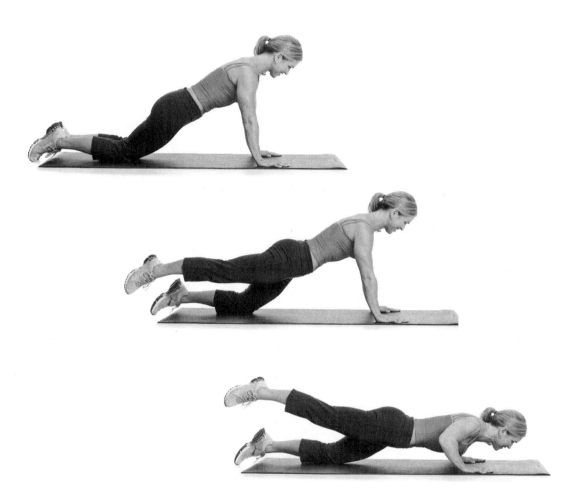

Assume a pushup position with your knees on the floor, your arms extended, and your hands on the floor beneath your shoulders, so your body forms a straight line from your head to your knees.

Lift one leg a few inches off the floor.

Bend your elbows to lower your chest toward the floor until your upper arms are parallel to the floor. Press back to the starting position, lowering your leg. Do the next rep with the opposite leg raised, and continue alternating legs until you complete the set.

DOUBLE-LEG STRETCH

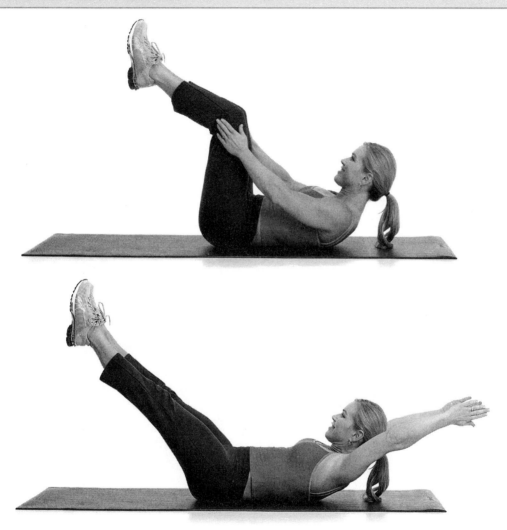

Lying faceup on the floor with your knees pulled in toward your chest, pull your navel toward your spine and contract your abs, raising your shoulders off the floor and extending your arms so your hands are beside your knees.

Inhale as you extend your arms and legs out at 45-degree angles, keeping your abs tight and lengthening through your limbs. Exhale as you bring your knees back toward your chest and return to the starting position.

PLATEAU-BUSTING LOG

Make photocopies of this log and use them to keep track of each and every one of the *Prevention*'s Shortcuts you take. Three to 5 days a week, you want to check off at least one Plateau Buster workout. Check off one of the cardio walking workouts every day, and do a second one at least 3 days a week. Also remember to give yourself extra credit for every 1-Minute Wonder and Lifestyle Shortcut you squeeze in.

	SUN	MON	TUES	WED	THU	FRI	SAT
Plateau Buster							
Workout A							
Workout B							
Workout C							
Cardio (see Chapter 4)							
Need for Speed							
Fast and Focused							
Strong and Steady							
Pyramid Power							
Rolling Hills							
Conquer the Mountain							
1-Minute Wonder							
Let Your Feet Do the Walking (page 36)							
Tap Your Toes! (page 76)							
Do "Invisible" Exercise (page 99)							
Multitasking Moves (page 149)							
Stealth Leg Slimmers (page 243)							

	SUN	MON	TUES	WED	THU	FRI	SAT
Sneaky Arm Shapers (page 295)							
Armchair Athletics (page 328)							
Lifestyle Shortcut							
Walk This Way (page 77)							
Take It Outside! (page 80)							
Take Action! (page 144)							
Just Say No (page 178)							
Use Flower Power (page 179)							
Think Positive! (page 180)							
Get Sleep! (page 190)							
Drink Up! (page 191)							
Laugh It Up . . . and Off (page 297)							
Hit the Pound (page 299)							
Hoop It Up (page 329)							
Step Up to the Plate (page 358)							
Live for the Future (page 360)							

Notes (goals, feelings, etc.): _____

_____

_____

_____

_____

_____

_____

FIND ANOTHER FINISH LINE

It's great to have a goal to get in shape. But it wouldn't be fair if I didn't warn you—sometimes that's not enough. Sure it feels great to hit your goal weight. You'll definitely be walking on air for a while when you finally squeeze into those jeans you thought were destined for Goodwill. But the problem with reaching your goal is, there's nothing left to shoot for. It's easy to lose motivation when you're working out every day to simply stay in place. That's why I encourage you to find a goal outside of yourself—something that will act as a carrot to keep you motivated to move and also instill in you a sense of accomplishment.

My favorite way to stay motivated is to sign up for an event like a 5-K run or charity bike ride. There's nothing like having a "race" on your calendar to motivate you to move. You'll notice I put the word *race* in quotation marks. That's because though many of these events are technically races, only about 10 percent of the participants are actually racing.

I remember years ago when my son was 8 and watching me run my first marathon. He was standing at mile 18, and by the time I cruised by, he'd watched literally a couple of thousand runners pass by. He looked at my husband and said sadly, "There's no way Mom is going to win this race." It's funny coming from a kid, but too often adults still view competition through the lens of winning. It's not like that. Most adults win a marathon simply by showing up! The majority of the participants are there for the camaraderie and personal challenge. They're everyday folks just like you and me. Most have jobs, mortgages, kids, and not much time. Some are thin and fit; most are average or even overweight. But they're there with smiles on their faces, enjoying an opportunity to celebrate physical movement. There's nothing like a free T-shirt, a goodie bag, and a raucous round of applause as you cross a finish line to make all your hard work feel very worthwhile. Try a race and I promise you'll be hooked for life.

The best part about these events is that you can exercise your altruism while working out your heart and lungs. There are thousands of charity walks, runs, bike rides, and triathlons across the country every year. You can Run for the Cure to raise money for breast cancer research. You can ride for multiple sclerosis. If there's a cause, there's an event to raise money for it. The quickest way to find what's going on in your area is to head to Active.com. Just search for events in your ZIP code and get started today.

SIZE MATTERS

Chances are you're pretty careful about what you eat. Most women who only have 10 or so pounds to lose are already pretty smart about avoiding fast food and generally eating a healthy diet. They just eat too much food, often without even realizing it, because America has a serious case of portion distortion.

Here are a few fast facts. Back in 1960, the standard hamburger was 1.5 ounces, and the standard pasta entrée 1½ cups. Today, the average portions for those and

CLEAN-EATING SHORTCUT
PAY ATTENTION TO PROTEIN

You may already be following the tips in Chapter 3 that ensure you not only shave your daily calorie intake but also eat a well-rounded diet. Since you're turning up your exercise intensity to blast through that weight loss wall, however, I want you to pay special attention to your protein intake.

New protein research from the University of Illinois at Urbana-Champaign reports that adding more fish, poultry, and lean meat to your diet will accelerate the benefits of your workout. In the study, researchers put 24 women on a fitness plan and asked half the group to eat about 9 ounces of high-quality protein a day, while the other half ate just 5 ounces of protein and twice as much carbohydrate-rich food. Though both groups consumed the same number of calories, the protein-only group lost 47 percent more weight than the carb group and 21.5 percent of their body fat, compared with 15 percent for the carb-heavy dieters. The researchers believe that protein helps work with insulin to better rebuild your muscles and rev metabolism.

Plan to have a little protein with every meal. Be creative. There is protein beyond chicken. Try soy foods and soybeans, kidney beans, and legumes and nuts, as well as fish, eggs, dairy, and meat. My favorite simple source of protein is peanut butter. I make it myself. Just pour a can of peanuts into the food processor and whip them around until smooth. The creamy result is absolutely delicious and incredibly healthy. Just remember not to overdo; it is calorie-dense, so a little goes a long way.

other foods have literally doubled! It's not uncommon to get 3 cups of pasta dished out in a serving bowl for just one person or to find yourself staring down a half-pound burger. Everything from chocolate bars to pizzas has increased in size. Experts estimate that we're eating hundreds of calories more than we need every single day simply because the sizes of everyday foods we're served at restaurants, cafeterias, and supermarkets have ballooned.

You would think it wouldn't matter—that if a 1.5-ounce burger was all we needed

LIFESTYLE SHORTCUT
JUST SAY NO

Most women I know suffer from yes-ism. "Mom, can you bake 3 dozen brownies for school tomorrow?" "Mrs. Jones, we need a volunteer for the Parks and Recreation Committee—could you do it?" "Honey, can you pick up the dry cleaning tomorrow?" "Debra, we're looking for someone to write a proposal for the McKinney Project. Can you do it?" Inside, your brain may be screaming, "No! No! No! No!" But when you open your mouth, all that comes out is "Uh, okay." "Sure." "No problem." "I'd love to."

It's natural to want to help your family, lend a hand to your community, and go above and beyond at work. But when we stretch ourselves too thin, something has to suffer, and I don't have to tell you that it's usually us! The stress of constantly taking on more than you want to do can compromise your health. Make a list of everything you contribute your energy to—charities, carpools, volunteering at school, sports, jobs, the works. Circle the things that make you feel good or you actually like doing. Consider dropping the rest (unless it's something you have to do, like a work project).

If you never turn down a task, people will expect you to always say yes, and the demands on you increase. By saying no once in a while, you send the message that your time is not limitless. Saying no may be very stressful initially, but you'll get over that stress within an hour or two. Saying yes to something you don't want to do can lead to weeks, even months of gnawing stress that wears you down and takes away from the things in life you love.

LIFESTYLE SHORTCUT
USE FLOWER POWER

Telling you to put some fresh flowers in your house may seem out of place in a fitness book, but I believe that the best physical results come when you take care of the whole person—mind, body, and spirit. That's why I'm a big fan of meditation, positive affirmations, and, yes, flowers. I will actually buy one less food item at the grocery store (something we don't really need) and substitute it with a bunch of fresh cut flowers; then I place them on my center island in the kitchen, where they make me happy all week long.

People have cultivated flowers for more than 5,000 years. We spend countless hours planting, weeding, fertilizing, arranging, painting, taking pictures of, and buying and selling flowers. And all they do is look pretty! Turns out, that's more than enough. Research shows that women who are given flowers enjoy a more positive mood for a full 3 days after they receive them. When flowers are presented to elderly people, they not only report having happier moods, but also perform better on memory tests. Flowers have an immediate and lasting effect on how we feel and how we react. Trying to change lifestyle behaviors and lose weight can be stressful. A vase or two of fresh cut flowers can make you feel better. Keep some in the kitchen and wherever you work out.

to feel satisfied 40 or 50 years ago, we would just take a few bites of a supersized burger and leave the rest on the plate. But we humans are designed to survive famines, so when food is plentiful, we feast! Studies show that people will eat 30 to 50 percent more food when they're served a large portion, and they don't necessarily feel more full or even stuffed. Again, it's because we are hardwired to eat abundant amounts of food when they're available so we'll have excess stores if our food supply disappears.

Unfortunately, as long as most Americans view Frisbee-size cookies and bucket-size soft drinks to be a "bargain," we can't expect food manufacturers to rightsize our portions anytime soon. It's up to us. The best way to start is to cut your restaurant portions in half (or order the appetizer version or a half portion when available), and

LIFESTYLE SHORTCUT
THINK POSITIVE!

Psychologists estimate that about 72 percent of our self-talk is negative or self-critical! Can you imagine how defeated you'd feel if someone else was putting you down all day? Well, your own berating can be just as damaging. We all have times when we feel defeated or tired, but the key to overcoming those spells is treating yourself to some positive affirmations. When I encounter stressful situations and am lacking self-confidence, I say to myself, "You can do it—you've done harder things than this before." I recount the numerous times I held a screaming baby for hours on end or comforted a broken-hearted 12-year-old, and I remind myself that I am powerful and that I am grateful and lucky to be able to face life's challenges. It may sound silly, but self-talk is one of the most powerful motivators. Try it for yourself.

ask for the other half to be wrapped up right away. Avoid buffets—research shows people eat 25 percent more in all-you-can-eat settings. Remember, most of the time, our eyes are much bigger than our stomachs, and I guarantee you'll be surprised at how much (or, in this case, little) food it takes to feel really satisfied.

PART 3

Prevention's Shortcuts to Shaping and Sculpting

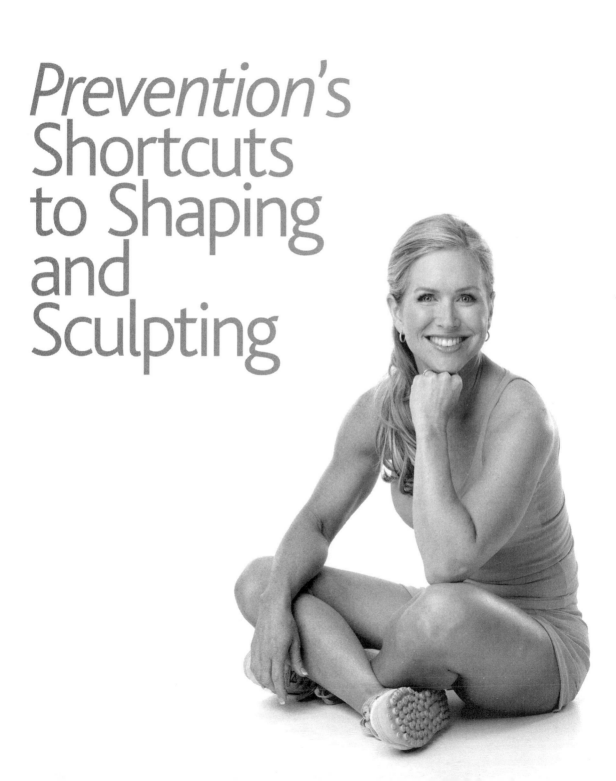

CHAPTER 7

Tone Your Trouble Spots in Short Order

'm a realist. As much as I want everyone to want to exercise to feel great and be healthy, I know that's not what drives the vast majority of women (or men!). You want to look good. Hey, it's absolutely human nature. And with the *Prevention*'s Shortcuts plan, you can make it happen in far less time than you ever thought possible!

I firmly believe that training programs are never one size fits all. So in this section, I've created four customized plans designed to tackle women's toughest toning challenges: stubborn belly bulges, heavy hips and thighs, bulging bottoms, and flabby arms. I've also included bonus programs for allover stiffness and achy backs.

My motto is exercise smarter, not harder, and *Prevention*'s Shortcuts body-sculpting plans do just that, to help you reshape and get results fast. The secret is building your workouts around your specific problem area. For instance, many women complain of belly bulges that won't budge no matter what they do. The *Prevention*'s Shortcuts approach tackles those untamable tummy muscles from the inside out. The deep transverse abdominal muscles become stretched and weak from underuse or pregnancy, so your belly may stick out no matter what your size. Through a special blend of core work, Pilates, and cardio to shed unwanted fat, you can pull those muscles taut and see results in as little as 2 weeks. Before you know it, you'll have the flat belly you've always dreamed of showing off.

Prevention's Shortcuts Success Story

"NOW I BURN EXTRA CALORIES INSTEAD OF CONSUMING THEM!"

Too many people think that in order to be fit, you need to dedicate hours in the gym. But if I wake up 30 minutes earlier, I can get in a quick workout in my own home and start the day with a sense of accomplishment and well-being. (Plus I only like to take one shower a day!)

Even when time is tight, I've found just 10 minutes can make a positive impact on my health. What works for me is taking 10 minutes to work a body area, like my arms, abs, or butt, during the late afternoon from 4:00 to 6:00 p.m. During this time, my kids are doing homework and I'm cooking dinner. I have noticed that this is also a big munching period for me. If I take 10 minutes to focus on exercising a body part, however, I have burned calories rather than consumed them. I am also less likely to munch because I don't want to ruin the hard work I just put in. It takes about 10 minutes to simmer sauce and cook pasta—perfect to squeeze in a small workout!

It's important that women take care of themselves. I know a lot of people depend on me. And I am more energetic, happy, and healthy because I choose to fit in chunks of time to exercise. I know I am a better mother, wife, and friend because I feel good about who I am and the example I am setting for my children.

Holly, 40

Whatever your special need, it's addressed in this section. And, as my philosophy goes, all you need is 10 minutes to take it on and finally put it in its place! You can incorporate any of these workouts into bonus Shortcut Slots while you're working toward your weight loss goals, since each toning program requires just 10 minutes three times a week. Then, once you've reached your goal weight using the programs in Part 2, you can devote yourself to the programs that follow to fix your particular problem areas while maintaining your weight with Chapter 4's cardio workouts.

Your *Prevention*'s Shortcuts workouts will be fast, and so will your results: You can slim saddlebags and thunder thighs in 8 weeks. Blast away cellulite, permanently, and get hot buns in as little as a month. Get the right to bare arms in 4 to 6 weeks. Become more limber and lithe in 3 weeks. And strengthen your back to feel and look strong and sexy in just 2 weeks.

10-SECOND WISDOM

"To keep the body in good health is a duty . . . otherwise we shall not be able to keep our mind strong and clear."

Buddha

YOGA POWER

The secret weapon in this section of the book: yoga poses, or asanas, that are low impact and excellent for increasing strength and stretching tight muscles. Why add these to the strength training exercises that work so well for burning fat? Because, like our hair and skin, our muscles and connective tissues become thinner and drier with age. With less fluid plumping them up, those tissues lose some of their elasticity. Stiff, rigid muscles constrict circulation by squeezing off your blood vessels. That means fewer nutrients can get into your muscles and less metabolic waste can get out. Eventually, hard knots called calcifications form, leaving you feeling about as flexible as frozen taffy.

But it doesn't have to be that way. Stretching is the solution. By extending your muscles through their full range of motion, you loosen the knots, boost circulation, and promote both the flow of oxygen and nutrients to your muscles and the elimination of built-up waste from those tissues. Each time you reach and bend, your body also gets the signal to produce more synovial fluid, the "oil" that lubricates your joints, so your shoulders, knees, hips, and ankles bend, twist, and rotate more smoothly. Just 10 minutes of stretching every day can easily restore decades worth of flexibility. And, hands down, my favorite way to stretch is yoga.

Yoga has been practiced around the world for more than 5,000 years as a way to increase range of motion, promote relaxation, and enhance self-awareness. It's been known to improve sleep, circulation, digestion, blood pressure, and cardiovascular function. Yoga—which is simply a series of standing, seated, and lying postures that stretch and strengthen your body and calm your mind—is not a religion, though it can be very spiritual. It's not a sport, though it can be very physical. In short, it is what you make of it.

Think you won't be able to do the poses because you're already pretty inflexible? If you have tight shoulders and haven't touched your toes in years, you're the perfect candidate. The goal isn't to be able to twist into a pretzel right away (if ever!) but rather to gradually and steadily improve from where you are now. There's no race, and it's no contest. Each pose can be adjusted to work with your personal abilities. As your practice continues, you can expect to be able to go deeper into each pose as you improve your range of motion.

And you will become more flexible—maybe dramatically so. In a study from the University of California, Davis, researchers found that men and women who practiced yoga twice a week improved their spinal flexibility—the ability to arch their backs—a whopping 188 percent! There's a saying that you're only as young as your spine, your body's "information superhighway" that delivers messages to your organs, muscles, and limbs. So if this study is any indication, yoga can make you a whole lot younger!

What's more, you'll become calmer. Each of your muscles is equipped with a stretch receptor that reports back to your brain about your overall level of tension. If you're walking around with your shoulders perpetually hunched up around your ears and your hamstrings wound tight as violin strings, your brain gets the message that you're under constant stress. By loosening those muscles, you send your brain a dramatically different message: Your body is relaxed, and, in turn, your brain relaxes.

Personally, I'm a type A, high-energy type of person. When stressed, I can get wound tight as a drum. For me, yoga is like personal therapy. With my muscles relaxed and my mind calm, I'm a better parent, friend, teacher, and spouse. That's why I like to start the day with yoga. It sets me up for a more even-tempered, balanced day. Other people like to practice at night to unwind, release tension, and sleep more peacefully.

Prevention's Shortcuts Success Story
"I LOVE THAT I CAN STAY FIT 10 MINUTES AT A TIME."

I own my own business and teach Sunday school, confirmation, and a women's group, all while chasing after four young daughters. So it's not unusual for me to find myself with limited time. But I want to be around for a long time and want to be able to do fun things with my daughters as they get older. I've found that exercise is the best way to lose weight and get in shape, so it's important that I keep moving—especially since as I get older, I find that it's harder to keep the weight off. I want to look the same as I did when I was 30, so finding time has been a priority.

I love the fact that if I have 10 minutes at any time of day, I can squeeze in a *Prevention*'s Shortcuts workout. I'll often do 10 or 20 minutes in the morning and more at night. The short workouts are very motivating because they go so fast, they leave you wanting to do more. I've also gotten my friends and family into the act. Some nights after work, we'll go for a family walk. And my daughters love to exercise with me. As soon as they see me in my workout clothes, they say, "When are we working out?" By shutting off the TV and getting active as a family, we're all happier and healthier.

Beth, 36

GO WITH THE FLOW

Don't worry if you don't look exactly like the yoga pictures in these chapters, especially at first. Everyone looks a little different on the outside when they practice yoga because our bodies are different. A friend of mine has what she calls freakishly long arms, so she can easily rest one hand on the floor in Triangle pose, whereas I can't.

But she might never be able to straighten those long arms in Cobra, as I can. What's important is what's happening inside—you're lubricating your joints, muscles, ligaments, and tendons and rejuvenating your spine and central nervous system.

No need for any special outfit or equipment (aside from maybe a mat if you have slippery floors)—just bare feet and clothes that allow you to comfortably move and stretch. Move into each pose slowly and purposefully, stretching only until you feel a slight "pull" or stretch in the muscle. You should feel tension relief, never pain.

And pay close attention to your breathing. *Pranayama*, or breathing deeply and fully through your nose and exhaling through your nose, is an essential component of yoga. To do it, flare your nostrils (instead of allowing them to suck in as they normally do during inhalation) to open your airway, and take a full deep inhalation until your lungs fill all the way. Then exhale through your nose, opening the back of your throat to create a tube. Pranayama keeps the breath internal, heating up from the inside out. Done properly, it can sound a little like Darth Vader.

Pranayama helps calm your mind and improves oxygen supply through the body, so you fully oxygenate and nourish every cell. As a bonus, yogic breathing can make you a better fat burner. Weight loss depends on raising metabolism and burning fat. You need oxygen to do both. The deeper you breath, the more oxygen you deliver to your cells to fire up their furnaces and burn fat.

10-SECOND WISDOM

"He who has health has hope. He who has hope has everything."

Arabian proverb

As you flow through the asanas, try to time your breathing with your movements, inhaling and exhaling as you initiate and move through the pose. Clear your mind and try to stay as present as possible, forgetting, just for 10 minutes, about unfinished business, dinner, bills, or other daily distractions. You'll be better able to attend to those things if you can put them aside while you do something for your body.

CHAPTER 8

Flat Stomach

Is a stubborn belly bulge your biggest body woe? You're in good company! More than half of Americans put "flatter stomach" at the top of their fitness wish list. Like millions of Americans, you probably wonder why you can do hundreds, if not thousands, of crunches and still see a flabby midsection when you look in the mirror.

The real deal is this: Crunches alone simply don't cut it. The way most people do them does more to strain your neck than challenge your core. Even done properly, this one-dimensional move works a single stomach muscle—the rectus abdominis, which runs from your ribs to your hips—leaving the rest of your midsection muscles out cold. The *Prevention*'s Shortcuts system offers a better way: Pilates-based exercise.

CORE POWER

Pilates is a system of precise, focused movements that are engineered to generate strength and power in your "core." The core is a big buzzword these days, but it's simply a shortcut way of talking about your obliques, the "twisting" muscles that wrap around the sides of your midsection; the rectus abdominis, or your six-pack muscle that runs the length of your front; the transversus abdominis, which is your deepest abdominal muscle and acts like a girdle to hold you upright and protect your spine (this one gets the most stretched during pregnancy); as well as the erector spinae muscles that run along your spine.

Developed by a German athlete named Joseph Pilates almost 100 years ago, Pilates

LIFESTYLE SHORTCUT
GET SLEEP!

Counting sheep may actually help take inches off your waist. Research shows that if you're sleep deprived, your body produces more stress hormones, which promote belly fat and also increase appetite. What's more, a new study shows that a sound night's sleep boosts levels of leptin, a hormone that works to suppress hunger.

To study the sleep-appetite connection, researchers at Laval University in Quebec tracked the sleep habits of 740 men and women for 10 years. As it turns out, the benefits of just *1 extra hour* of sleep are astonishing! The researchers found that women who got 6 to 7 hours of sleep were 11 pounds heavier (men fared even worse—16½ pounds heavier) than those who slept 7 to 8 hours a night. Blood tests revealed that short sleepers had levels of leptin 80 percent below those who got a full night of shut-eye. Turn off the TV an hour before bedtime, unwind with a good book, and get some sleep. It's good for your waist.

Even though I know it in theory, I did my own personal experiment with sleep recently. Due to some insane scheduling at the time, I was getting about 5 hours of sleep a night, sometimes even less on the weekends. I found myself unable to concentrate, which was no surprise. But more interestingly, I was constantly wanting to eat. My body was craving any form of energy it could get. And since I wasn't giving it sleep, it was demanding food. So I changed my work hours and got my much-needed sleep. Guess what? The cravings vanished—literally overnight!

had been a mainstay of dancers and athletes in this country for decades before hitting the mainstream fitness industry and becoming a household term during the past 10 or 15 years. Done regularly, Pilates can tighten your core for a firm, flat appearance. What's more, the moves in this section also protect you from the back injuries and pain that drive so many people to doctors' offices every day. They improve your posture, which by itself can make you look 5 pounds slimmer. Most important, these moves improve strength, coordination, balance, flexibility, and joint mobility. You'll sit and stand straighter, walk taller, move with more ease and grace, and, yes, finally be able to zip up those old Calvin Kleins.

Not all the exercises in this chapter are strictly Pilates, but all are grounded in the basic concepts of both Pilates and yoga (another discipline rooted in precise, focused movement). The program is also extremely time efficient. You will feel the effects of these moves immediately and, depending on your body type, may see results in as little as 2 weeks.

DIET ALONE WON'T DO IT—BUT FOOD COUNTS!

Before you read any farther, let's make sure this chapter is really where you should be. Too many clients who complain about "flabby abs" don't really have flabby abs; they have fat over their abs. This isn't meant to be insulting, simply educational. Many people still don't recognize that you can't "spot reduce" and that all the situps and crunches in the world won't burn belly fat. So you might actually have the most ripped rectus abdominis in the world, but unless you lose that layer of fat on top through diet and exercise, no one will ever see it.

The best way to lose belly fat is a combination of healthy eating and active living. In fact, though you can drop pounds just through dieting, belly fat isn't likely to

LIFESTYLE SHORTCUT
DRINK UP!

Water is your weight loss ally. Your body needs to be properly hydrated to metabolize fat and keep your systems running optimally. Water is the best fluid for the job. When University of North Carolina researchers reviewed the eating habits of nearly 5,000 Americans, they found that those who drank about 7 cups of water a day ate 200 fewer calories than those who drank less than a glass a day. Water-phobes were also more likely to chow down more high-fat foods and drank twice as many soft drinks as clear-liquid lovers.

What's more, water can kick-start your metabolism. German researchers recently discovered that about 2 cups of ice water can raise metabolism by 30 percent for 90 minutes. I keep a water bottle with me at all times—in my car and in my bag. I sip on it all day long. If I get bored of plain water, I drink flavored water to inspire me to keep sipping. Propel by Gatorade is one of my favorites. Grab an icy cold bottle of fresh fluid and sip away the weight.

budge without exercise, according to a study from Wake Forest University in Winston-Salem, North Carolina. In a 5-month study, researchers there had a group of women either cut 400 calories a day from their diets but not exercise, or exercise enough to burn 400 calories. At the end of the study, both groups lost about the same amount of weight—23 pounds. But the daily exercisers trimmed 16 percent of their belly fat, while those who dieted alone saw no fat cell shrinkage in their midriff. Why? Because cardio exercise triggers your body to convert abdominal fat to fuel.

That said, there's no denying that how much you eat determines the width of your waistline. Trimming a few pounds can be as simple as taking a few less bites, literally. Experts find that all those extra nibbles, from sampling the goodies in your co-worker's candy dish to picking at leftovers after dinner, can add up to 500 calories a day. Consider other people's plates (and sweets jars) off-limits. And take leftovers straight to the fridge or the trash, if they won't keep. You may hate to waste food. But it sure beats "waisting" it.

QUELL STRESS

Uncontrolled stress can boost belly fat in two ways. It increases levels of the hormone cortisol, which studies show sends fat to the abdominal region. And since eating reduces tension, stress can drive you to overeat, especially the sugary, high-calorie comfort foods.

Exercise helps burn off stress hormones like cortisol and, over time, makes you more resistant to the effects of stress. If your stress levels are still in the red, try a few minutes of meditation every day. It doesn't have to be spiritual or religious or New Agey. Just sit down, close your eyes, and do a little self-reflection. Think about what is good in your life, and take a moment to feel grateful for what you have. Sit in silence and clear your mind. Or sit and listen to some soft music that makes you feel good. Read a book of favorite poems. If Americans would take just a few moments a day to be still and reflect, we'd be a calmer, happier, more satisfied nation.

If there is something specific that is worrying you, then do something about it. No matter how big your worry, action is the best cure. It makes you feel in control. If you're worried about your job, have lunch with your supervisor and ask her what you could be doing better—or start keeping your eyes open for another job. Worried about your kids? Get more involved in their lives, or, if they've left the nest and gone

CLEAN-EATING SHORTCUT
GO WITH THE GRAIN

Fiber is a flat belly's best friend. It helps fill you up, so you feel satisfied with less food. It keeps things moving, so you're less likely to get bloated and constipated. And it helps fight heart disease, diabetes, and cancer. Yet many Americans still get only half of the 20 to 35 grams of fiber they should be eating every day. Plant foods are by far your best source of fiber. Fruits and veggies are loaded with it. Another important source is whole grain foods.

The USDA recommends that we all consume three or more servings of whole grains every day. "Whole grain" means that the food contains the entire edible portion of any grain, whether it be wheat, oats, barley, or rye. The closer you get to the original form of the grain, the better.

To make it easier for consumers to identify whole grain foods, the Whole Grain Council has come up with a series of stamps for whole grain products. When you see a stamp that says "100% Whole Grain Excellent Source," it means the food contains a full serving and that all grains are whole grains. A stamp that says "Whole Grain Excellent Source" means the product contains a full serving of whole grain. "Whole Grain Good Source" means the food delivers a half serving of whole grain. Shoot for three full servings a day.

---

out on their own, stay close to them by e-mailing or instant messaging. It's amazing how many worries can be put by the wayside when we bring them out into the open, talk about them, and take action. You are the master of your own domain. Believe it, and take control.

CELEBRATE YOUR SHAPE

Finally, in your quest to have a flat belly, don't forget that women are also meant to have curves. If you look at an anatomical illustration of the abdominal muscles, you'll notice how the top half has horizontal bands running through, creating a "six-pack" effect, but the lower half is one smooth band of muscle running down to the pelvis. So even if you lost every ounce of fat (which is physically impossible to do . . . and live to tell about it), you would still have a small curve in your lower belly. It's the beauty of the female shape. It's okay to want to tighten up your midriff and lose the "pooch." But learn to love your natural curves.

As detailed in the workout descriptions for these moves, you should begin each exercise by contracting the transversus abdominis first. Never push your abs out. Instead, draw or scoop them in toward your spine. When I say (again and again) to draw your navel toward your spine, that is intended to activate your transversus abdominis and protect your back.

Do one workout from this chapter 3 to 5 days a week. If you feel highly motivated or have extra time, you can do more than one workout in a day, but that's not necessary. I've provided three different abdominal workouts—A, B, and C—and you can choose whichever one(s) you like, though I recommend mixing them up rather than doing the same one every time. I also recommend plenty of cardio—at least one of the Chapter 4 workouts every day, plus a second one of those workouts 3 to 5 days a week. And whenever possible, try a Lifestyle Shortcut, a 1-Minute Wonder, or any of the *Prevention*'s Shortcuts workouts from any other chapters in the book that strike you as fun and interesting. Use the log on page 216 to keep track of what you've done each day.

WORKOUT A

Do two sets of 12 to 15 repetitions for each exercise except for Child's Pose, which you should hold for 20 to 30 seconds. You can either do both sets of a single exercise consecutively or do one set of every exercise and then repeat.

Pilates Crunch

Bicycle

Double-Leg Stretch

Swimming

Spinal Balance and Crunch

Child's Pose

PILATES CRUNCH

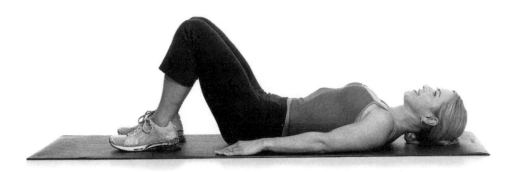

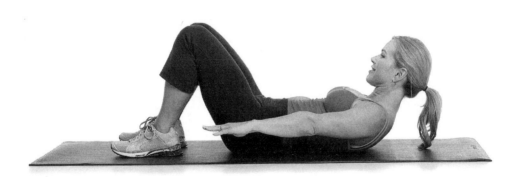

Lie faceup on the floor with your knees bent, your feet hip-width apart and flat on the ground, and your arms at your sides, palms on the floor.

Visualize sliding your rib cage to your pelvis as you pull your navel toward your spine, contract your abs, and sequentially roll your head, shoulders, and upper back off the floor. As you perform the move, lengthen through the back of your neck and tuck your chin slightly toward your chest, while keeping your arms parallel to the floor. Lower back to the starting position. This is the difference between mindlessly crunching and really pulling in and activating your deep transversus abdominis to make your core muscles work.

BICYCLE

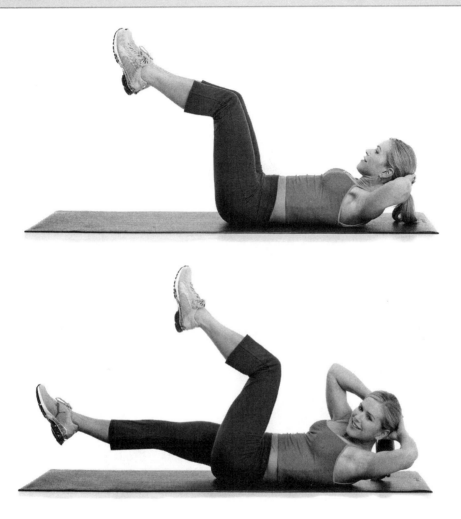

Lie faceup on the floor with your hips and knees bent to about 90-degree angles and your abs tight to protect your lower back. With your hands behind your head, carefully lift your head and shoulders off the floor.

Pull your left knee toward your chest while extending your right leg straight out, parallel to the floor. At the same time, lift and twist your torso to bring your right elbow toward your left knee. Return to the starting position, then repeat on the other side.

DOUBLE-LEG STRETCH

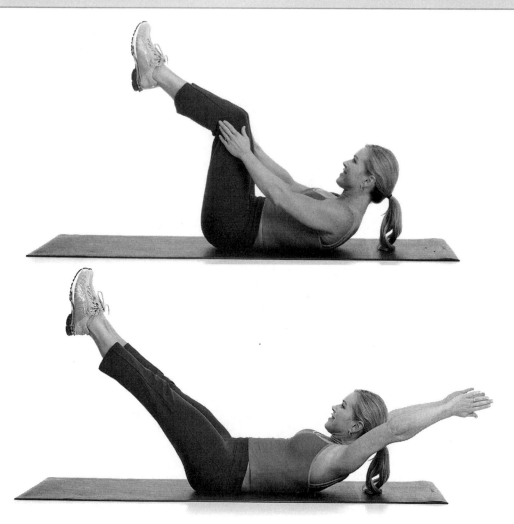

Lying faceup on the floor with your knees pulled in toward your chest, pull your navel toward your spine and contract your abs, raising your shoulders off the floor and extending your arms so your hands are beside your knees.

Inhale as you extend your arms and legs out at 45-degree angles, keeping your abs tight and lengthening through your limbs. Exhale as you bring your knees back toward your chest and return to the starting position.

SWIMMING

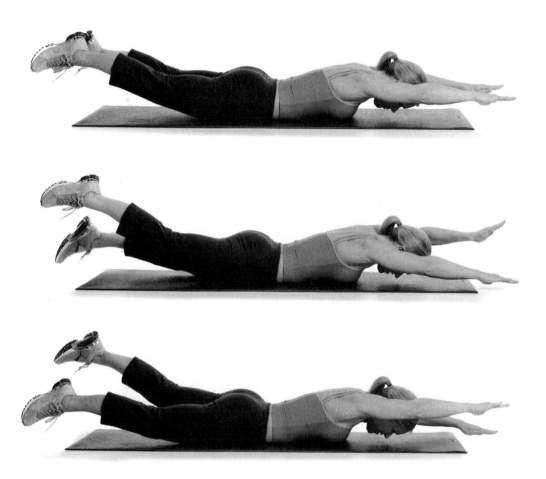

Lie facedown on the floor with your arms extended out in front of you and your legs extended back. Lift your limbs up off the ground and keep your abs tight. Point your fingertips and toes to create a long spine.

Flutter opposite arms and legs simultaneously, while breathing smoothly and steadily.

SPINAL BALANCE AND CRUNCH

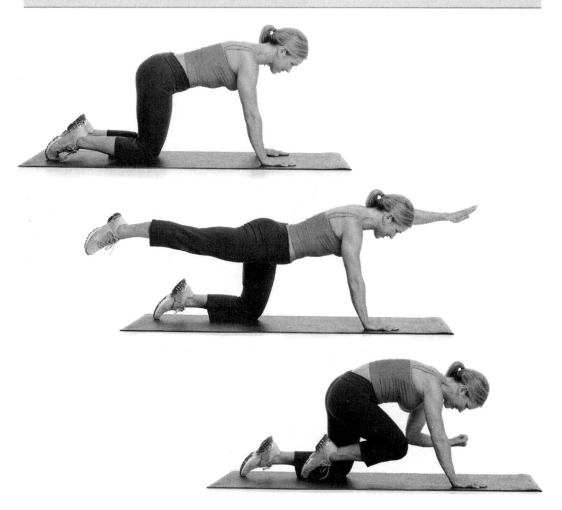

Kneel on all fours, with your hands directly beneath your shoulders and your knees directly beneath your hips. Keep your back straight and your head in line with your spine.

Draw your navel toward your spine and simultaneously raise your left arm and right leg, extending them in line with your back so your fingers are pointing straight ahead and your toes are pointing back. Hold for 2 seconds.

Then contract your abs and draw your left elbow and your right knee together, beneath your torso. Complete a full set, then switch sides.

CHILD'S POSE

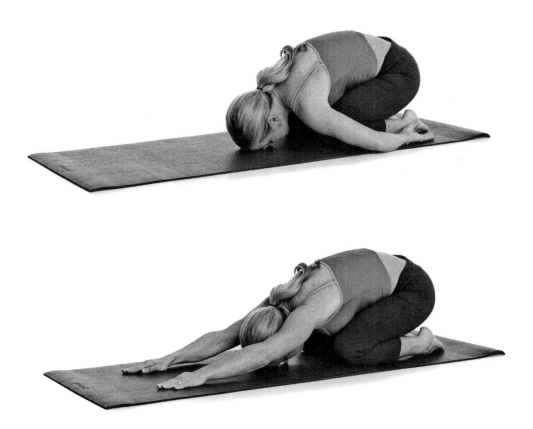

Kneel and then sit with your hips back on your heels. Lower your upper body down over your lap and rest your forehead on the floor. Rest your arms at your sides, palms facing up.

Or you can extend your arms straight out in front of you, reaching and spreading your fingers. Relax your neck, face, and shoulders as you take deep, slow breaths.

This pose is relaxing and rejuvenating. It relieves tension in your neck, shoulders, and spine.

WORKOUT B

Do two sets of 12 to 15 repetitions for each exercise except for Child's Pose, which you should hold for 20 to 30 seconds. You can either do both sets of a single exercise consecutively or do one set of every exercise and then repeat.

Half Roll-Back

Full-Body Roll-Up

Bicycle

Side Hip Lift

Swimming

Child's Pose

HALF ROLL-BACK

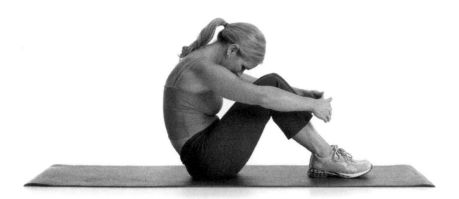

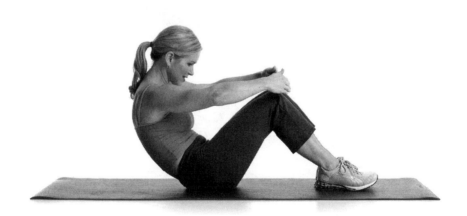

Sit on the floor with your knees bent and your feet and knees separated slightly. Pull your navel toward your spine and curl your spine forward so your torso is bent over your legs in a C shape. Reach your arms forward, with your shoulders relaxed.

Exhale and, maintaining a C shape with your spine, roll halfway back by tucking your tailbone and lowering vertebrae by vertebrae. Inhale and pull your abs even closer toward your spine. Then exhale and contract your abs to return to the starting position. Maintain a rounded spine throughout the movement.

FULL-BODY ROLL-UP

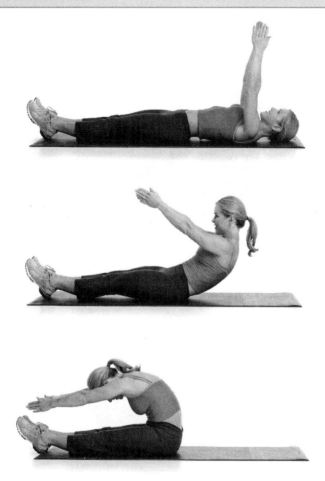

Lie faceup on the floor with your arms relaxed and extended straight up. Pull your navel toward your spine to engage your abdominal muscles as you inhale and stretch your arms upward.

Exhale, lengthen the back of your neck, tuck your chin toward your chest, and, keeping your navel pulled toward your spine, curl forward with your arms extending in front of you. Visualize leading with the top of your head to create a C curve, curling forward until you are reaching for your toes. Inhale as you stay rounded.

Begin reversing direction, uncurling your body. Exhale as you continue to "drip" your spine back to the floor, one vertebrae at a time, slowly lowering back to the starting position.

BICYCLE

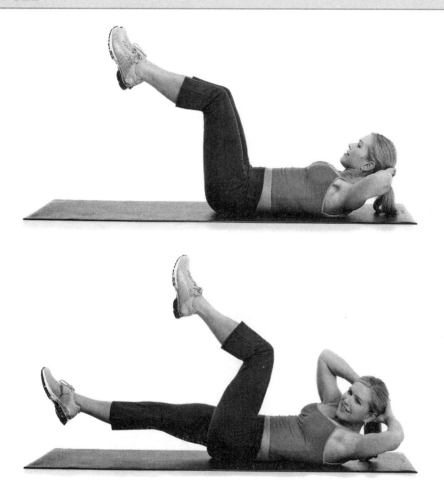

Lie faceup on the floor with your hips and knees bent to about 90-degree angles and your abs tight to protect your lower back. With your hands behind your head, carefully lift your head and shoulders off the floor.

Pull your left knee toward your chest while extending your right leg straight out, parallel to the floor. At the same time, lift and twist your torso to bring your right elbow toward your left knee. Return to the starting position, then repeat on the other side.

SIDE HIP LIFT

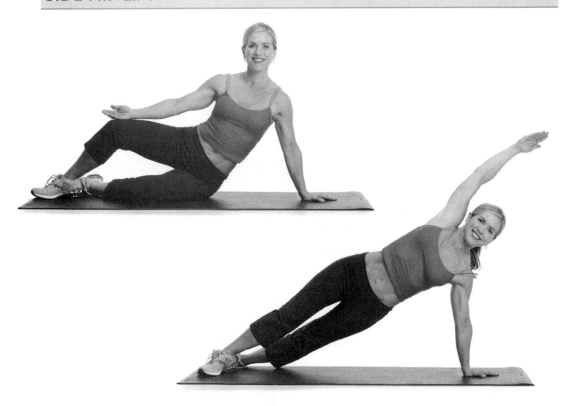

Sit on your left hip with your legs extended to your right, knees slightly bent. Cross your right foot just in front of your left. Place your left hand on the floor, in line with your left shoulder, for support. Extend your right arm and place your right hand on your right knee, palm facing up.

Pull your navel toward your spine, contract your obliques, and lift your hips off the floor while extending your right arm overhead, so your body forms a straight diagonal line. Then, without bending your left arm, lower your hips and right arm back to the starting position.

Complete a set, then repeat on your other side.

If you're a beginner, keep your left knee on the floor.

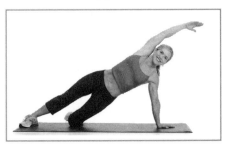

SWIMMING

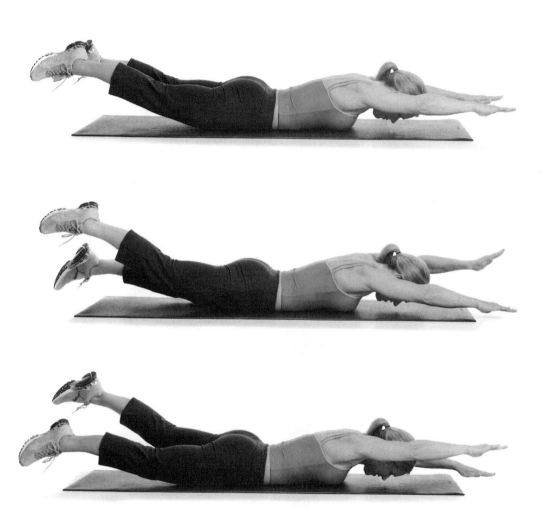

Lie facedown on the floor with your arms extended out in front of you and your legs extended back. Lift your limbs up off the ground and keep your abs tight. Point your fingertips and toes to create a long spine.

Flutter opposite arms and legs simultaneously, while breathing smoothly and steadily.

CHILD'S POSE

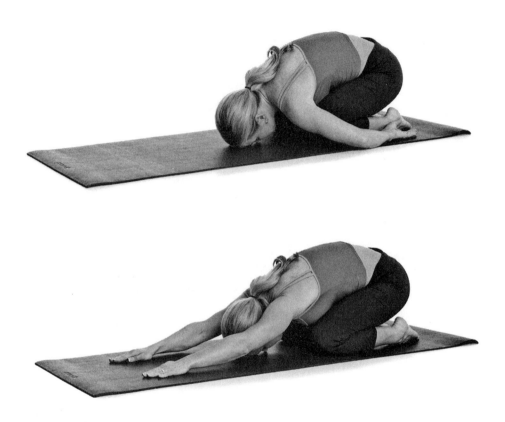

Kneel and then sit with your hips back on your heels. Lower your upper body down over your lap and rest your forehead on the floor. Rest your arms at your sides, palms facing up.

Or you can extend your arms straight out in front of you, reaching and spreading your fingers. Relax your neck, face, and shoulders as you take deep, slow breaths.

This pose is relaxing and rejuvenating. It relieves tension in your neck, shoulders, and spine.

WORKOUT C

Do two sets of 12 to 15 repetitions for each exercise except for Child's Pose, which you should hold for 20 to 30 seconds. You can either do both sets of a single exercise consecutively or do one set of every exercise and then repeat.

Balancing Side Twist

Pilates Crunch

Straight-Leg Reverse Curl

Double-Leg Stretch

Spinal Balance and Crunch

Child's Pose

BALANCING SIDE TWIST

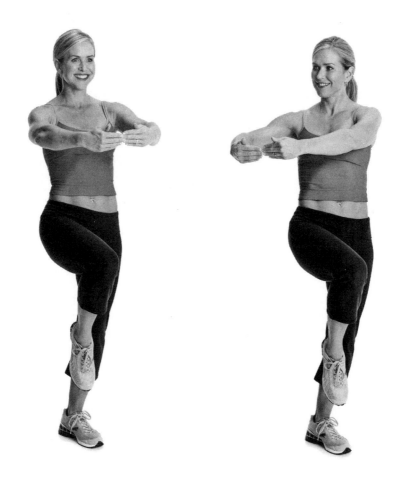

Stand tall on your left leg, with your right leg lifted at a 90-degree angle straight out in front of you. Extend your arms in front of you at shoulder height and curve them in slightly as though you were hugging a beach ball.

Pulling your navel toward your spine and keeping your hips square and facing forward, turn your torso to the right as far as you comfortably can without turning your hips. Wrap your rib cage to the side as though wringing out a washcloth. Return to the starting position. Complete a set before switching legs and performing the move to the left.

PILATES CRUNCH

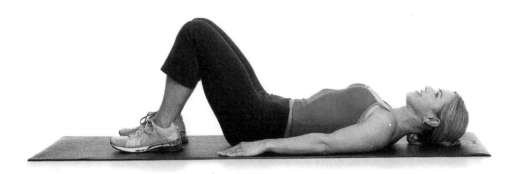

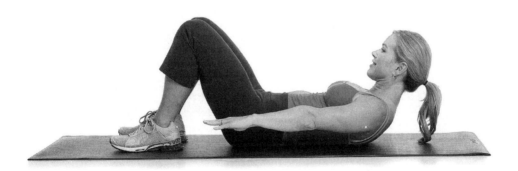

Lie faceup on the floor with your knees bent, your feet hip-width apart and flat on the ground, and your arms at your sides, palms on the floor.

Visualize sliding your rib cage to your pelvis as you pull your navel toward your spine, contract your abs, and sequentially roll your head, shoulders, and upper back off the floor. As you perform the move, lengthen through the back of your neck and tuck your chin slightly toward your chest, while keeping your arms parallel to the floor. Lower back to the starting position. This is the difference between mindlessly crunching and really pulling in and activating your deep transversus abdominis to make your core muscles work.

STRAIGHT-LEG REVERSE CURL

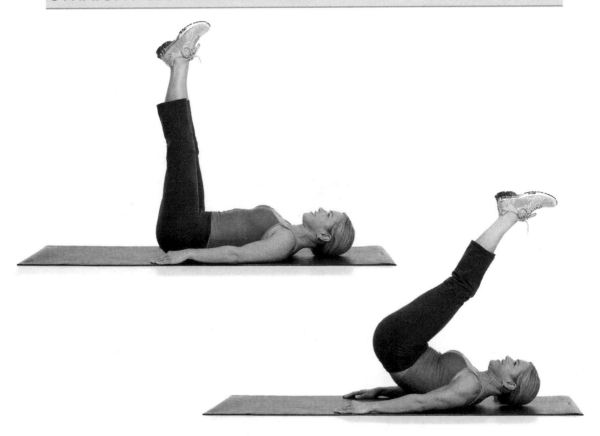

Lie faceup on the floor with your arms at your sides, legs extended into the air at a 90-degree angle to your tailbone on the mat.

Draw your navel toward your spine to scoop your abs and curl your hips off the floor so your feet move slightly over your head. Hold for a moment, then slowly lower back to the starting position.

If your hamstrings are tight, keep your knees slightly bent throughout this exercise.

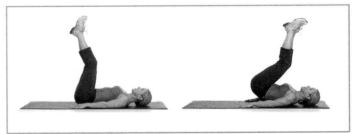

DOUBLE-LEG STRETCH

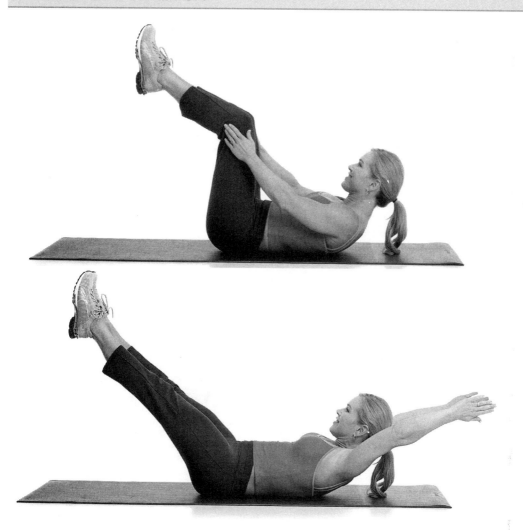

Lying faceup on the floor with your knees pulled in toward your chest, pull your navel toward your spine and contract your abs, raising your shoulders off the floor and extending your arms so your hands are beside your knees.

Inhale as you extend your arms and legs out at 45-degree angles, keeping your abs tight and lengthening through your limbs. Exhale as you bring your knees back toward your chest and return to the starting position.

SPINAL BALANCE AND CRUNCH

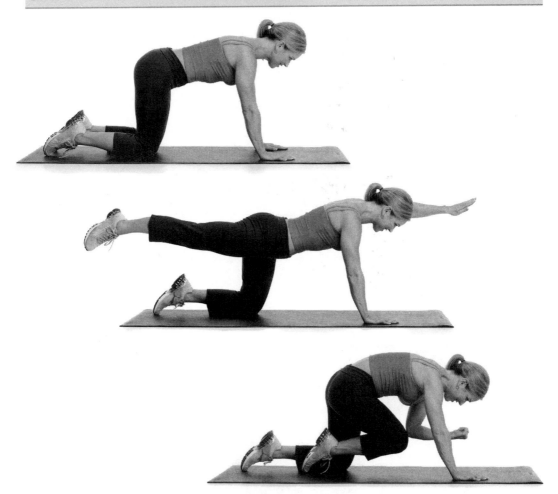

Kneel on all fours, with your hands directly beneath your shoulders and your knees directly beneath your hips. Keep your back straight and your head in line with your spine.

Draw your navel toward your spine and simultaneously raise your left arm and right leg, extending them in line with your back so your fingers are pointing straight ahead and your toes are pointing back. Hold for 2 seconds.

Then contract your abs and draw your left elbow and your right knee together, beneath your torso. Complete a full set, then switch sides.

CHILD'S POSE

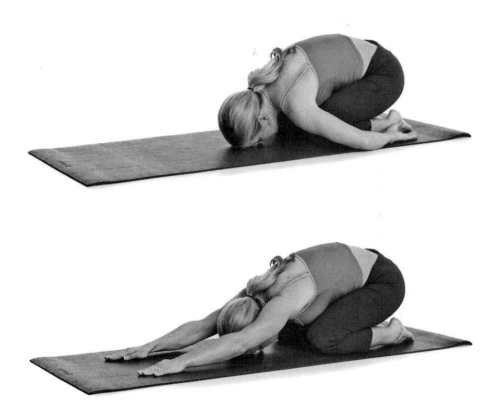

Kneel and then sit with your hips back on your heels. Lower your upper body down over your lap and rest your forehead on the floor. Rest your arms at your sides, palms facing up.

Or you can extend your arms straight out in front of you, reaching and spreading your fingers. Relax your neck, face, and shoulders as you take deep, slow breaths.

This pose is relaxing and rejuvenating. It relieves tension in your neck, shoulders, and spine.

FLAT STOMACH LOG

Make photocopies of this log and use them to keep track of each and every one of the *Prevention*'s Shortcuts you take. Three to 5 days a week, you want to check off at least one Flat Stomach workout. Check off one of the cardio walking workouts every day, and do a second one at least 3 days a week. Also remember to give yourself extra credit every time you squeeze in a 1-Minute Wonder, Lifestyle Shortcut, or *Prevention*'s Shortcut from other chapters.

	SUN	MON	TUES	WED	THU	FRI	SAT
Flat Stomach							
Workout A							
Workout B							
Workout C							
Cardio (see Chapter 4)							
Need for Speed							
Fast and Focused							
Strong and Steady							
Pyramid Power							
Rolling Hills							
Conquer the Mountain							
1-Minute Wonder							
Let Your Feet Do the Walking (page 36)							
Tap Your Toes! (page 76)							
Do "Invisible" Exercise (page 99)							
Multitasking Moves (page 149)							
Stealth Leg Slimmers (page 243)							
Sneaky Arm Shapers (page 295)							

	SUN	MON	TUES	WED	THU	FRI	SAT
Armchair Athletics (page 328)							
Lifestyle Shortcut							
Walk This Way (page 77)							
Take It Outside! (page 80)							
Take Action! (page 144)							
Just Say No (page 178)							
Use Flower Power (page 179)							
Think Positive! (page 180)							
Get Sleep! (page 190)							
Drink Up! (page 191)							
Laugh It Up . . . and Off (page 297)							
Hit the Pound (page 299)							
Hoop It Up (page 329)							
Step Up to the Plate (page 358)							
Live for the Future (page 360)							
Other *Prevention*'s Shortcuts							

Notes (goals, feelings, etc.): _____

_____

_____

_____

_____

_____

_____

CHAPTER 9

Lean, Toned Thighs

It's no secret that women are constantly waging war with their legs—especially their thighs. According to a poll by the National Women's Health Resource Center, a full 36 percent of us report that our bottom halves are usually where fat goes to stay. That's simply a biological fact: Nature pads excess fat around our thighs to ensure we have some fuel reserves to ride out a pregnancy and feed hungry babies during times of famine.

Given that anatomical fact, the best way to trim your thighs is simply to use them. Walk, run, ride a bike, skip, take the stairs—anything to get off your seat and move your lower half. The biggest muscles in your body are in your legs. When you challenge them by hiking, hill climbing, or riding a bike on an incline, you use *lots* of oxygen and burn mega calories.

To firm your thighs and create some sleek, sexy curves, add strength training. When we talk about toned thighs, we really mean strong, fit legs! By taking your legs through a full range of motion and challenging them from every angle, you can sculpt shapely legs you'll love.

SADDLEBAGS AND THE UNSUNG SUPPORTERS

Most women think of their legs strictly in terms of thighs and calves. But your thighs are actually made of four distinct muscle groups. At the front of the thigh is your quadriceps, which is the muscle that straightens your leg. The back thigh muscle is the hamstring, which you use to bend your legs. On either side are your abductors on the outside (including some of your glute muscles), which you use to pull your leg away from your body and your adductors on the inner thigh, which bring the legs back toward your body. We use our quads and hamstrings all day long as we walk, climb stairs, and get in and out of chairs. But unless you play tennis, ski, or do some other sport with lots of side-to-side motion, chances are your abductors and adductors go underused. That's why so many women complain of flabby inner thighs or "saddlebags" around their hips.

The *Prevention*'s Shortcuts workouts in this chapter are carefully crafted to focus on all the major muscles in the legs. Lunges and squats are the core of any good leg workout because they target all the muscles in the thighs, especially the quadriceps. But I also chose moves like ballet sweeps and leg circles, which zero in on the outer thighs, and pliés, which shape up the stubborn inner thigh area. Together these routines will give you fabulously strong legs, from every angle, in just 4 to 6 weeks.

10-SECOND WISDOM

"Successful people aren't just lucky. They work hard and prepare themselves so they are ready when opportunity knocks."

The following workouts target your quads and hamstrings as well as outer and inner thighs. For sleek, sexy legs, do one workout 3 to 5 days a week. If you feel highly motivated or have extra time, you can do more than one workout in a day, but that's not necessary. I've provided three different workouts—A, B, and C—and you can choose whichever one(s) you like, though I recommend mixing them up rather than doing the same one every time. I also recommend plenty of cardio—at least one of the Chapter 4 workouts every day, plus a second one of those workouts 3 to 5 days a week. And whenever possible, try a Lifestyle Shortcut, a 1-Minute Wonder, or any of the *Prevention*'s Shortcuts workouts from any other chapters in the book that strike you as fun and interesting. Use the log on page 240 to keep track of what you've done each day.

WORKOUT A

For each exercise, do two sets of 12 to 15 repetitions (for each leg, where appropriate). You can either do both sets of a single exercise consecutively or do one set of every exercise and then repeat.

Simple Squat

Curtsy Lunge

Bridge "Bun" Lift

Prone Hamstring Curl

Side-Lying Leg Circle

SIMPLE SQUAT

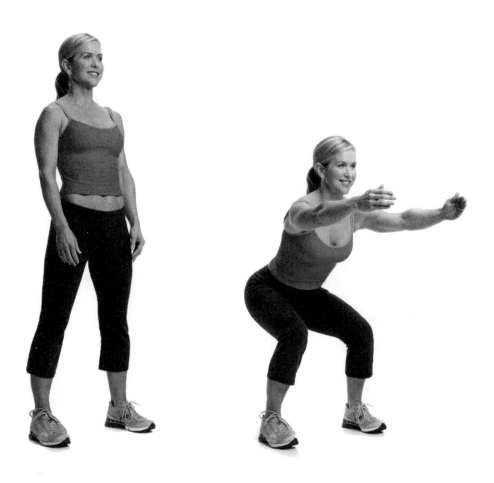

Stand with your feet hip-width apart, toes facing forward, abs tight, and arms at your sides.

Bend your knees to lower your body into a squat position, going as low as you can but no farther than knees bent to 90 degrees. Pretend you are sitting back into a chair—stick out your buns, keep your chest lifted and spine long, and extend your arms out in front of you—and keep your knees above your ankles. Push through your heels and squeeze your buns to rise back to the starting position.

CURTSY LUNGE

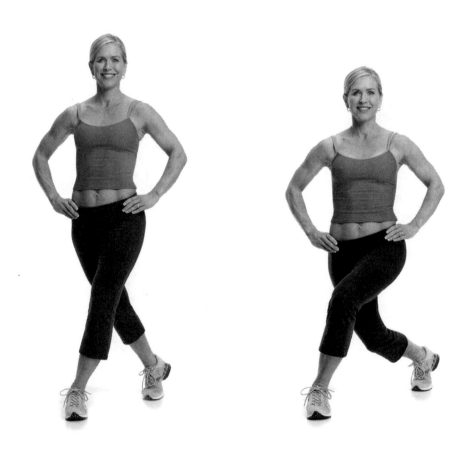

Stand with your feet hip-width apart, hands on your hips. With your right leg, take a giant step back and to the left so that if you were standing on a clock, facing 12, your right foot would end up at the 8 o'clock position.

Keeping your back straight and your head up, bend your knees to lower your hips toward the floor until your left thigh is parallel to the ground. Press into your left leg to rise back to the starting position. Complete a full set, then switch sides.

BRIDGE "BUN" LIFT

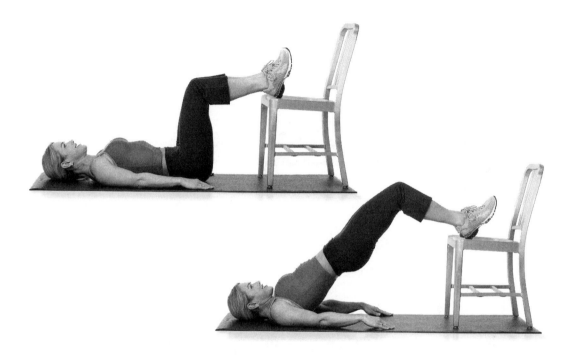

Lie on the floor and place your heels hip-width apart on the edge of a chair seat (or on a step, if a chair is too high), arms down by your sides, palms down.

Keeping your hips square to the ceiling and your navel pulled toward your spine, press into your

heels, squeeze your buns, and lift your hips toward the ceiling so your body forms a straight line from your knees to your shoulders. You can use your hands for balance but not to push yourself up. Lower back to the starting position.

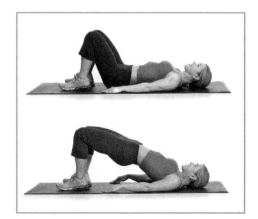

Beginners can try this first without a chair, feet on the floor.

PRONE HAMSTRING CURL

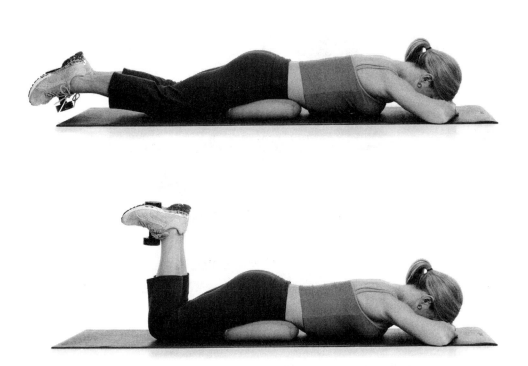

Lie facedown with a small pillow under your hips. Extend your legs and hold a dumbbell between your feet. Bend your arms in front of your face and rest your forehead on your hands for comfort.

Slowly bend your knees to curl the weight up and in toward your buns while pressing your hips against the floor. Then slowly straighten your legs to lower back to the starting position.

SIDE-LYING LEG CIRCLE

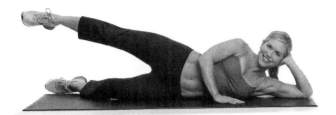

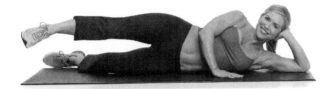

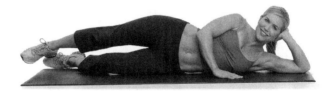

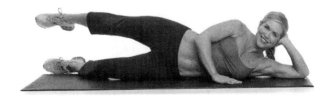

Lie on your left side, supporting your head with your left hand, or resting it on your left forearm, if that is more comfortable. Bend your left leg slightly for support and rest your right hand on the floor near your chest. Point your right toes and lift your right leg about 45 degrees, keeping your abs tight and your hips stacked and facing forward.

Initiating the movement from your hips, make small clockwise circles with your right big toe. Draw six circles. Then reverse the direction and draw six more. Repeat with the opposite leg.

WORKOUT B

For each exercise, do two sets of 12 to 15 repetitions (for each leg, where appropriate). You can either do both sets of a single exercise consecutively or do one set of every exercise and then repeat.

Simple Squat

Stationary Lunge

All-Fours Glute Lift

Ballet Leg Sweeps

Plié Calf Raise

SIMPLE SQUAT

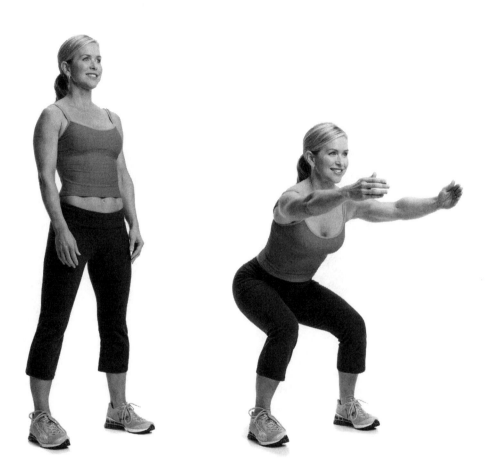

Stand with your feet hip-width apart, toes facing forward, abs tight, and arms at your sides.

Bend your knees to lower your body into a squat position, going as low as you can but no farther than knees bent to 90 degrees. Pretend you are sitting back into a chair—stick out your buns, keep your chest lifted and spine long, and extend your arms out in front of you—and keep your knees above your ankles. Push through your heels and squeeze your buns to rise back to the starting position.

STATIONARY LUNGE

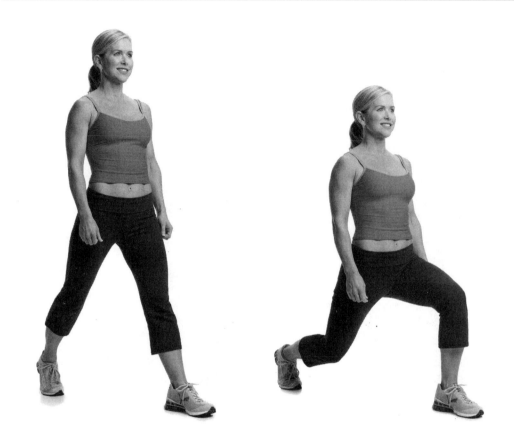

Stand in a split stance: front foot flat on the floor, back heel raised.

Bend both knees and lower into a lunge, keeping your front knee directly above the ankle and your back knee pointing down at the floor. Keep your abs tight, chest lifted, and spine long. Lower your body only as far as is comfortable. Don't bend your knees more than 90 degrees. Squeeze through your buns to raise yourself back up.

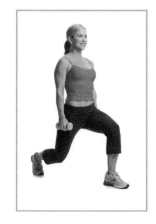

For a more advanced exercise, hold hand weights. Do a full set, then switch legs.

ALL-FOURS GLUTE LIFT

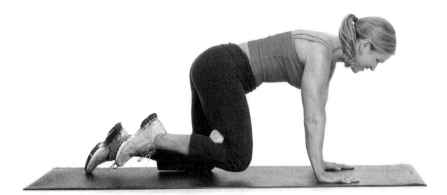

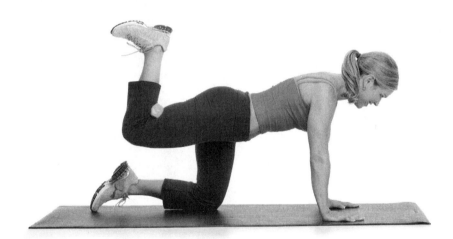

Get down on all fours, shoulders above wrists, hips above knees. Place a light weight behind one knee and bend your leg to hold it in place. Flex your foot. Tighten your abs and flatten your back.

Squeeze your butt muscles to lift your weighted leg until it is level with your hip. Lower back to the starting position. Repeat for a full set, then switch sides.

BALLET LEG SWEEPS

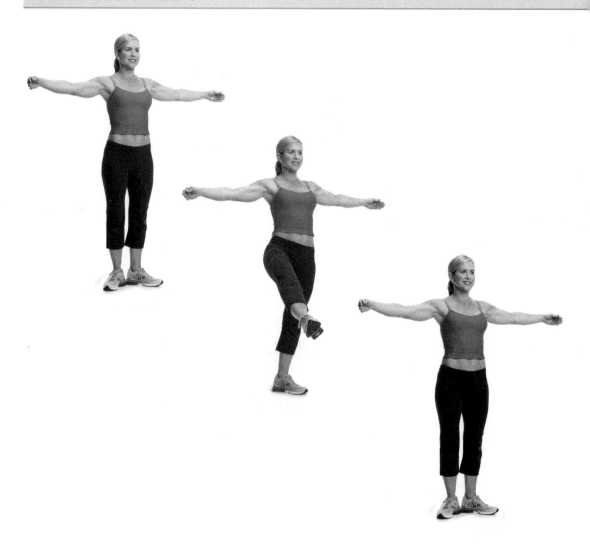

Stand straight with your arms extended out to the sides (or with your hands on the back of a chair for balance), feet together, and toes and knees turned out to the sides as far as comfortably possible.

Keeping your torso and hips steady, extend one leg, toes pointed, straight out in front of you as far as possible without shifting your hips.

Return to the starting position.

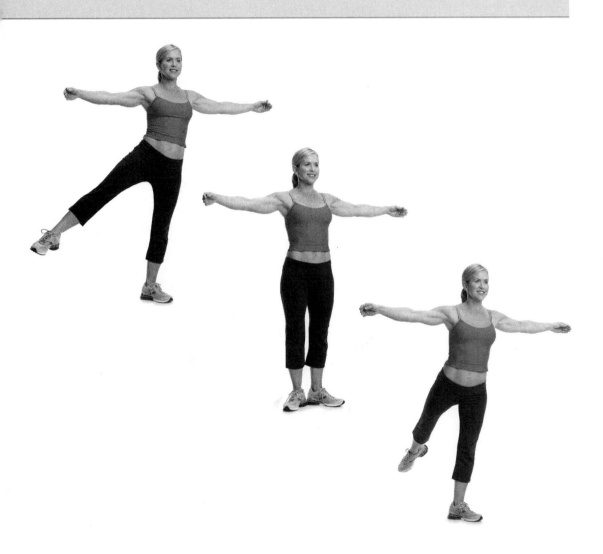

Using the same technique, extend your leg out to the side, then to the back, and to the side again to complete one rep. Finish a set, then switch legs.

PLIÉ CALF RAISE

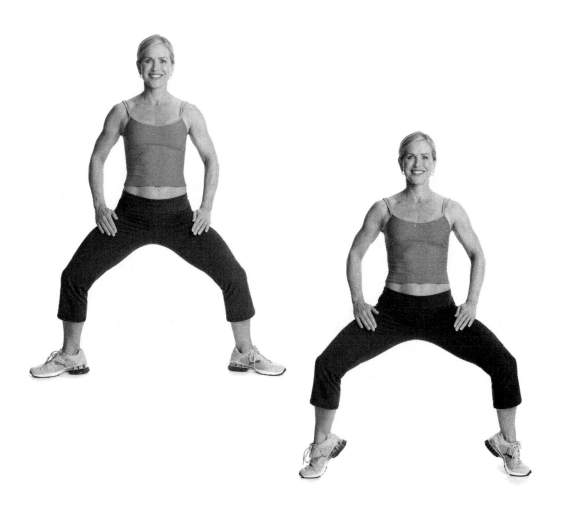

Stand with your feet farther than shoulder-width apart, heels facing in and toes pointing out. Place your hands on your upper thighs right below your hips. Keeping your back straight, begin to plié by bending your knees to send them toward your toes, tucking your tailbone underneath you as if you were sliding down an imaginary wall.

Hold this plié as you lift your heels and rise onto the balls of your feet. Then lower your heels, pressing them down. Continue to hold the plié while lifting and lowering your heels to complete the reps.

WORKOUT C

For each exercise, do two sets of 12 to 15 repetitions (for each leg, where appropriate). You can either do both sets of a single exercise consecutively or do one set of every exercise and then repeat.

Ballet Leg Sweeps

Plié

Crescent Lunge

Prone Hamstring Curl

Side-Lying Leg Circle

BALLET LEG SWEEPS

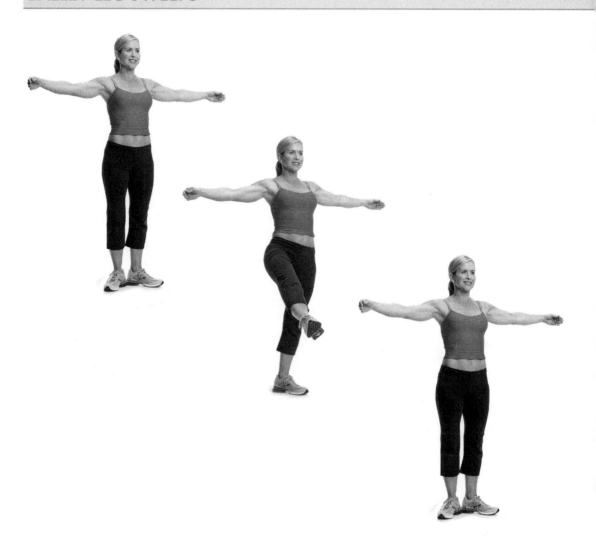

Stand straight with your arms extended out to the sides (or with your hands on the back of a chair for balance), feet together, and toes and knees turned out to the sides as far as comfortably possible.

Keeping your torso and hips steady, extend one leg, toes pointed, straight out in front of you as far as possible without shifting your hips.

Return to the starting position.

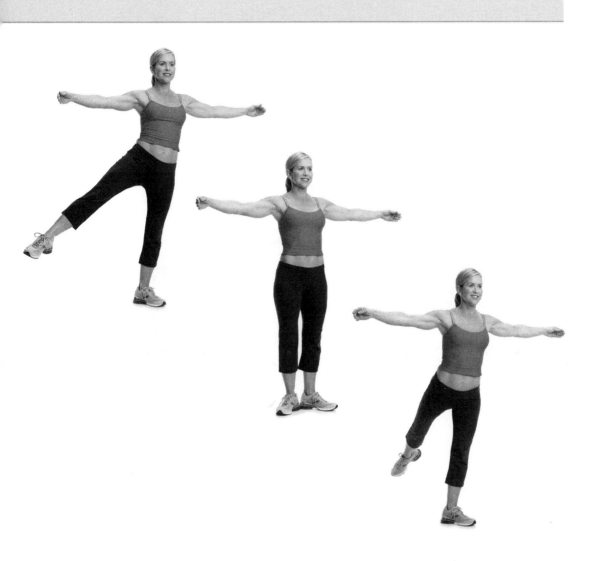

Using the same technique, extend your leg out to the side, then to the back, and to the side again to complete one rep. Finish a set, then switch legs.

PLIÉ

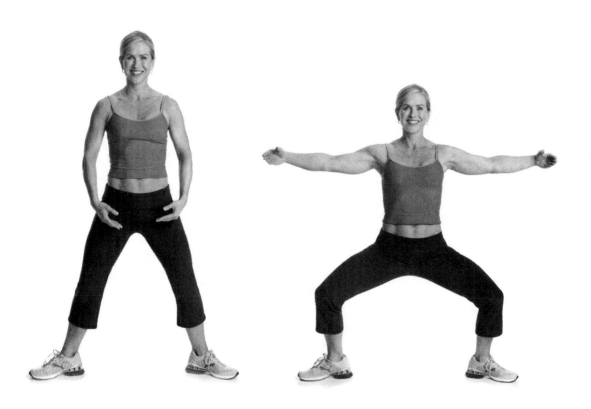

Stand with your feet farther than shoulder-width apart, toes pointing out.

Raise your arms straight out to the sides, palms facing forward. Keeping your back straight, extend your knees over your toes and tuck your tailbone underneath you as if you were sliding down an imaginary wall. Then press into your feet and squeeze your buns to rise back to the starting position.

For a more advanced exercise, deepen your range of motion, trying to get your thighs parallel to the floor.

CRESCENT LUNGE

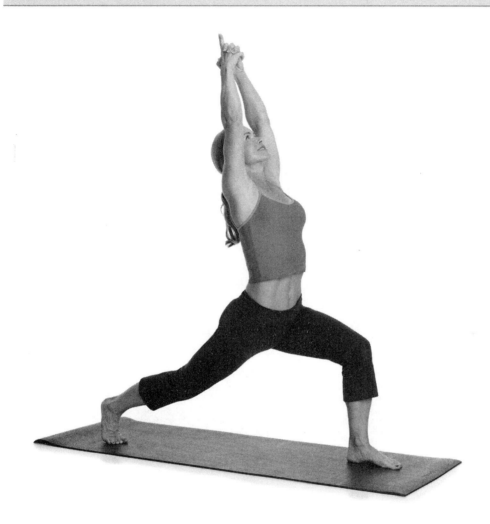

Stand in a lunge position with your right leg forward and bent 90 degrees, your right knee directly over your right ankle. Lower your left knee toward the floor, lifting your breastbone and raising your arms overhead. Clasp your hands together so your index fingers point toward the sky, and look upward, bending backward slightly. Breathe smoothly as you relax into the stretch. Switch sides.

This low lunge is great for opening your hips and stretching your quads.

PRONE HAMSTRING CURL

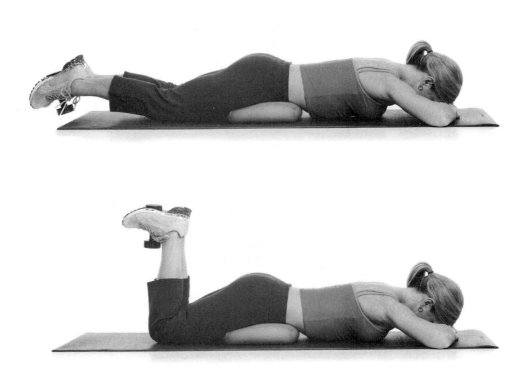

Lie facedown with a small pillow under your hips. Extend your legs and hold a dumbbell between your feet. Bend your arms in front of your face and rest your forehead on your hands for comfort.

Slowly bend your knees to curl the weight up and in toward your buns while pressing your hips against the floor. Then slowly straighten your legs to lower back to the starting position.

SIDE-LYING LEG CIRCLE

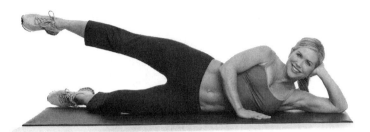

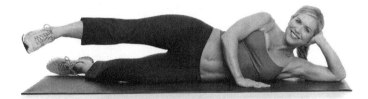

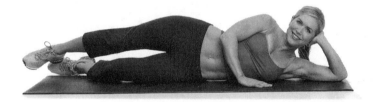

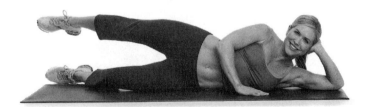

Lie on your left side, supporting your head with your left hand, or resting it on your left forearm, if that is more comfortable. Bend your left leg slightly for support and rest your right hand on the floor near your chest. Point your right toes and lift your right leg about 45 degrees, keeping your abs tight and your hips stacked and facing forward.

Initiating the movement from your hips, make small clockwise circles with your right big toe. Draw six circles. Then reverse the direction and draw six more. Repeat with the opposite leg.

LEAN, TONED THIGHS LOG

Make photocopies of this log and use them to keep track of each and every one of the *Prevention*'s Shortcuts you take. Three to 5 days a week, you want to check off at least one Lean, Toned Thighs workout. Check off one of the cardio walking workouts every day, and do a second one at least 3 days a week. Also remember to give yourself extra credit every time you squeeze in a 1-Minute Wonder, Lifestyle Shortcut, or *Prevention*'s Shortcut from other chapters.

	SUN	MON	TUES	WED	THU	FRI	SAT
Lean, Toned Thighs							
Workout A							
Workout B							
Workout C							
Cardio (see Chapter 4)							
Need for Speed							
Fast and Focused							
Strong and Steady							
Pyramid Power							
Rolling Hills							
Conquer the Mountain							
1-Minute Wonder							
Let Your Feet Do the Walking (page 36)							
Tap Your Toes! (page 76)							
Do "Invisible" Exercise (page 99)							
Multitasking Moves (page 149)							
Stealth Leg Slimmers (page 243)							

	SUN	MON	TUES	WED	THU	FRI	SAT
Sneaky Arm Shapers (page 295)							
Armchair Athletics (page 328)							
Lifestyle Shortcut							
Walk This Way (page 77)							
Take It Outside! (page 80)							
Take Action! (page 144)							
Just Say No (page 178)							
Use Flower Power (page 179)							
Think Positive! (page 180)							
Get Sleep! (page 190)							
Drink Up! (page 191)							
Laugh It Up . . . and Off (page 297)							
Hit the Pound (page 299)							
Hoop It Up (page 329)							
Step Up to the Plate (page 358)							
Live for the Future (page 360)							
Other *Prevention*'s Shortcuts							

Notes (goals, feelings, etc.): _____

_____

_____

_____

_____

_____

_____

STEP-BY-STEP

The easiest way to use your legs more is to walk more, all the time, everywhere. Whether you're tidying up the house or walking the mall, every step counts. For weight loss, you should aim to accumulate about 10,000 steps a day, about 5 miles' worth. If you literally forget to get up and move—meaning you sat down at the computer "just to check e-mail" at 9:00 a.m. and suddenly it's lunchtime—I recommend investing in a pedometer.

These devices strap onto your waistband (there are some you can even slip in your pocket or purse) and keep a running tally of every step. You can buy one for less than $25 at major sporting goods stores. They're wildly popular in Japan and parts of Europe and are growing increasingly popular among fitness enthusiasts in the United States.

If gadgets aren't your thing, don't sweat it. There are plenty of ways to track your progress. An average city block is about 250 steps, and there are 2,000 steps (8 blocks) to every mile. So if you walk the dog around your neighborhood or run errands on foot, it's easy to figure how far you've gone. Or you can use time as your guide. Most people take about 100 to 130 steps (depending how fast you're walking) per minute while bustling about their day.

LIFESTYLE SHORTCUT
APPRECIATE YOUR OWN BRAND OF BEAUTY

Fitness magazines are a wonderful source of new moves and inspiration. But don't make the mistake of getting caught up in trying to look just like the models that grace their pages. For one, most of these women look great because it's their job to work out and look beautiful. The typical woman has many other things—including her own job!—to focus on. What's more, never underestimate the power of makeup and good lighting. Believe me, I know firsthand! Even those models couldn't look as good as they do without all that professional styling, lighting, and camera work. Besides, you can't accomplish anything positive when you're feeling negative emotions like envy and jealousy. So go ahead and feel inspired to look lean and beautiful in your own way, but don't lose yourself by always wishing you looked like someone else.

1-MINUTE WONDER
STEALTH LEG SLIMMERS

Even if you're forced to spend much of your work-week chained to your desk or standing around, there are ways to challenge your hips and thighs without anyone suspecting you're exercising. The following are some of my favorite sneaky leg slenderizers.

Play flamingo. Tone your hips and thighs whenever you're stuck standing in line. Simply lift your right foot and place it against the calf of the grounded leg. Contract your left quad and glute for balance while reaching the crown of your head to the ceiling to stand as tall as possible. Hold for 10 to 30 seconds, then switch sides. If that gets easy, try lifting yourself up on the ball of your grounded foot while balancing.

Scissors sit. Push back from your desk and sit at the edge of your office chair with your back straight. Extend your legs straight in front of you and lift your feet off the floor as high as comfortably possible, opening your feet about hip- to shoulder-width apart. Point your toes and turn your legs out slightly. Keeping your legs extended, open and close them like scissors, crossing the left ankle over the right, then opening up and immediately crossing the right over the left. Keep switching quickly 30 to 40 times.

Sneak in squats. Squats are some of the best moves for thigh toning. And what is a squat but sitting down and standing up, something you do dozens of times every day? Sneak in some exercise every time you get in and out of a chair by making a conscious effort to not use your hands to assist you. You'll be surprised how challenging it is—and how strong your legs become.

Do curbside calf raises. Anytime you're standing around near a step or a curb, you have the perfect opportunity to do some calf raises. Simply stand on the edge of the step with your heels hanging off the edge. Let them drop as low as comfortably possible, then raise up onto the balls of your feet. To add to the challenge, try one leg at a time.

Drop your heels. High heels may make your legs look long and lean, but they do very little to actually help tone them. In fact, a Turkish study found that high heels slow your walking speed about 6 percent. What's more, because your heel is elevated, you lose the "push off" phase on every stride, so you actually use a third less leg muscle per step—not to mention that walking long distances in high heels wreaks havoc on your knees. Opt for low-heeled shoes when walking around town, and save the stilettos for special occasions when you'll just be sitting around looking good!

CLEAN-EATING SHORTCUT
BE A BIG DIPPER

To prevent unwanted pounds from creeping on your lower half, you need to keep an eye out for unseen calories. One of the top sources in the American diet is sauces! Restaurant cooks have a habit of drowning everything in dressings, sauces, melted cheese, butter, and oil, so even a reasonable portion can contain hundreds of hidden calories.

The easiest way to avoid getting "sauced" is to ask for everything on the side. Order salad dressings, dipping sauces, and cream sauces on the side. Then take your fork and dip the tines in the sauce before stabbing your food. I am the Queen of Dipping! That way, I'm sure to get just the right amount of flavor, as well as a big savings in calories and fat.

TRY SOME NEW WHEELS!

If you want to sculpt your thighs without taxing your knees, get a pair of in-line skates. Anyone who has ever roller-skated or ice-skated will find this activity a snap to learn, and it's a fun way to spend a Saturday afternoon. In-line skating, or Rollerblading, was all the rage about 10 years ago and is now enjoying a resurgence in popularity, with lighter, faster skates that are easier on the ankles.

Rollerblading scorches more than 800 calories an hour and is far less jarring than other high-intensity sports like jogging—plus it doesn't feel like a high-intensity sport! Because you use your outer and inner thigh muscles as well as your quads and hamstrings, in-line skating targets and tones your thighs better than almost any other sport. If you're nervous about stopping and turning, just practice in an empty parking lot before taking your skates for a spin through your local park or on a pedestrian path. When beginning, always wear wrist guards for protection, in case you fall. Each season, I practice stopping a few times, then go gingerly the first time out to get back into the swing of it. Rollerblading is by far my favorite summertime leg shaper!

CHAPTER 10

Beautiful Booty

The human body is the most highly adaptive "machine" on the planet, and no body part is better evidence of that than the backside! Our glutes have the potential to be the strongest muscles in our bodies, giving us the power to lift children, carry heavy bags of groceries up stairs, and run, jump, and play. The more we use them, the more powerful they become.

Unfortunately, the opposite is just as true. The more we sit, the softer our seats. With all the time we spend parked in bucket seats, office chairs, recliners, and restaurant booths, most of us have spent years developing pretty cushy tushes. Worsening the situation, like our thighs, our buns are one of Mother Nature's favorite places to store "fuel reserves" in case of famine. So along with soft muscles, you likely also have excess fat wreaking havoc on your bottom line.

For shaping the backside, lunges and squats are your main ticket for success. However, it's also important to burn the fat that covers the beautiful muscle underneath. That's why my *Prevention*'s Shortcuts Beautiful Booty workouts mix quick-burst and plyometric (hopping and jumping) moves with glute strengthening exercises to get your heart rate up and burn extra calories while still using the buns to do most of the work. The result will be a tighter, firmer backside that helps you ski down mountains, swim across lakes, and live your life more energetically.

FAT BY ANY OTHER NAME

No booty chapter would be complete without a discussion of cellulite. And the truth is that 90 percent of women, even the skinniest ones, have some dimples back there.

CLEAN-EATING SHORTCUT
QUASH CRAVINGS

Nothing can derail healthy eating habits more quickly than powerful cravings for something decidedly unhealthy. Cravings can hit out of the blue, but most of the time they're associated with something specific like stress or PMS. Indulging yourself once in a while is perfectly okay, but if cravings start becoming daily occurrences, you need to find a way to calm them. One tried-and-true way is distraction: Leave the kitchen and do something else. If that's not possible, try these craving quenchers.

Pop some pickles. Strong-tasting foods like olives, pickles, and hot peppers are overwhelming to your tastebuds, which experts say cuts cravings off at the pass.

Gum up the works. I chew bubble gum when I can't stop eating—it keeps my jaw going, and it's sweet!

Satisfy your hunger. When cravings strike, ask yourself if you're actually hungry. If so, make a deal with yourself to first satisfy your hunger with some healthy food, and then you can have a taste of whatever you're craving if you still want it.

Brush your teeth. Ever notice how nothing tastes very good after you brush your teeth? Next time you're trying to avoid the box of chocolate bars you bought from a school fundraiser, give your pearly whites a quick cleaning. A swish of mouthwash or popping a mint can have the same effect.

What happens if these strategies don't work

It's not some mysterious condition that requires pricey medical procedures (in fact, liposuction can make it worse) or fancy pills or supplements. It's not the product of trapped "toxins" or poor circulation. It's one thing and one thing alone: fat. It just looks different because of how it's arranged.

Everyone has strands of connective tissue that separate fat cells into compartments and connect fat tissue to the skin. In women, these strands are arranged in a honeycomb-like pattern, which allows excess fat to bulge, creating the unsightly bumps and dimples we all dread. Men have smoother fat deposits back there because their connective tissue runs in a crisscross pattern, which prevents bulging. Even if you never had cellulite when you were young, it's not uncommon to have patches

and you find yourself slipping? Remember that we all blow it sometimes. We polish off the leftover pasta before we can lock it away in the Tupperware, or we find ourselves staring at an empty ice cream container when all we wanted was a taste. Too often women take a single episode of overeating and turn it into 3 days of dietary havoc. No one ever got fat from one overindulgence. Don't beat yourself up about it. It'll only lead to feelings of failure and increase your odds of overeating again.

Don't punish yourself by skipping meals or starving yourself for the rest of the day, either. That almost guarantees you'll overdo it the next time you sit down with a plate of food. Instead, shrug it off and get right back on track. There's always tomorrow. Remember, it's what you do most of the time—not those few occasions you fall off the wagon—that determines your success.

While you're at it, please put to rest the all-or-nothing attitude about sweets once and for all. No more reasoning that "I blew it with one cookie, so I might as well have six!" Choosing to eat one cookie isn't blowing it. I know I couldn't live without an oatmeal-raisin cookie every so often. The key to good, sustainable health is to make your lifestyle centered on choices, not on whether or not you "cheat."

appear later in life, as our skin gets thinner and those strands of connective tissue thicken with age. Plus, many of us add a few extra pounds in our adult years. Because fat is soft and squishy, it doesn't hold skin taut the way muscle does.

The good news is that because cellulite is fat, you can conquer it with *Prevention's* Shortcuts. As you burn more calories and work your glutes from every angle, you reduce the underlying fat stores and replace lost muscle tissue to give the area a more toned, taut appearance. As you strengthen your hamstrings and glutes, you tighten the honeycombs, making it less likely for the fat to push through.

Research confirms it. In a study of 16 women strength training 3 days a week, exercise physiologist Wayne Westcott, PhD, found that after just 8 weeks, the women lost over 3 pounds of fat, added 2½ pounds of muscle, and shed almost 1½ inches from their hips. When they took an ultrasound test of their legs, they found that the cellulite was literally disappearing. The women shrunk the lumpy fat layer by 1.3 millimeters and increased their lean, smooth muscle tissue by almost 2 millimeters. Expensive potions may give you a temporary improvement in appearance, but the lift from exercise is permanent.

The following workouts will firm and lift your buns for a better rear view in 4 to 6 weeks. Do one workout from this chapter 3 to 5 days a week. If you feel highly motivated or have extra time, you can do more than one workout in a day, but that's not necessary. I've provided three different Beautiful Booty workouts—A, B, and C—and you can choose whichever one(s) you like, though I recommend mixing them up rather than doing the same one every time. I also recommend plenty of cardio—at least one of the Chapter 4 workouts every day, plus a second one of those workouts 3 to 5 days a week. And whenever possible, try a Lifestyle Shortcut, a 1-Minute Wonder, or any of the *Prevention*'s Shortcuts workouts from any other chapters in the book that strike you as fun and interesting. Use the log on page 268 to keep track of what you've done each day.

WORKOUT A

Do 12 to 15 repetitions of each of the strength exercises, and do each Cardio Quick Takes exercise for 1 minute. Then repeat the whole workout.

Split Jump

Simple Squat

Lighting the Torch

Reverse Lunge/Lateral Raise

Ski Hop

Bridge "Bun" Lift

SPLIT JUMP

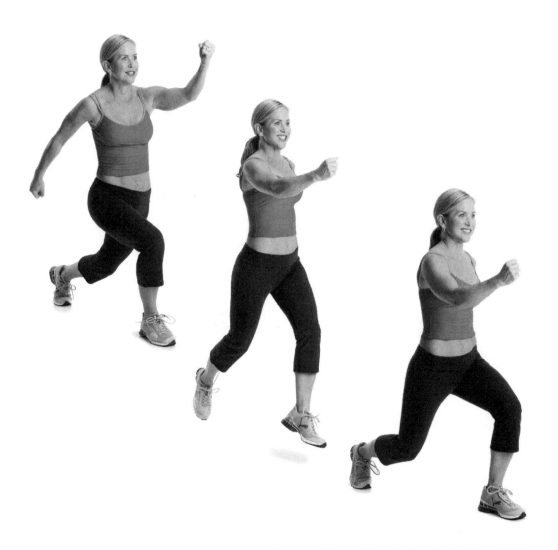

Begin in the basic lunge position. Leap straight up and switch legs in the air, landing with bent knees into a lunge with the opposite leg in front. Do this Cardio Quick Take for 1 minute.

SIMPLE SQUAT

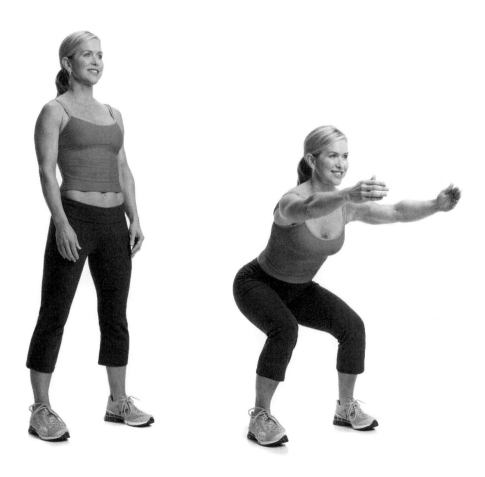

Stand with your feet hip-width apart, toes facing forward, abs tight, and arms at your sides.

Bend your knees to lower your body into a squat position, going as low as you can but no farther than knees bent to 90 degrees. Pretend you are sitting back into a chair—stick out your buns, keep your chest lifted and spine long, and extend your arms out in front of you—and keep your knees above your ankles. Push through your heels and squeeze your buns to rise back to the starting position.

LIGHTING THE TORCH

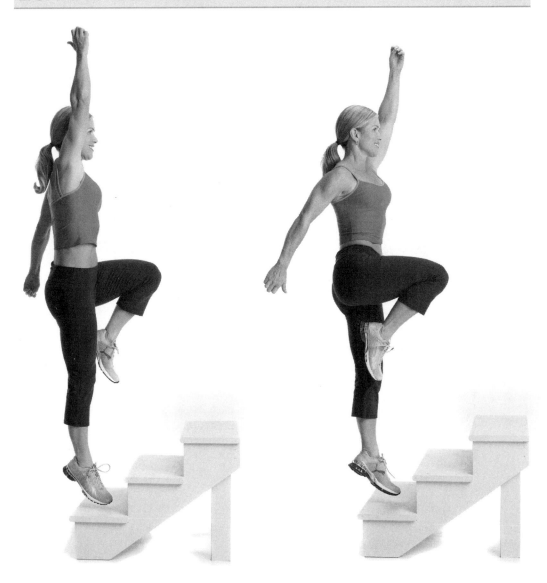

Stand on the floor in front of a staircase, and step onto the bottom step with your right foot while simultaneously lifting your left knee and right arm. Step back down to the floor with your left foot and then your right, then immediately step up with your left foot while raising your right knee and left arm.

REVERSE LUNGE/LATERAL RAISE

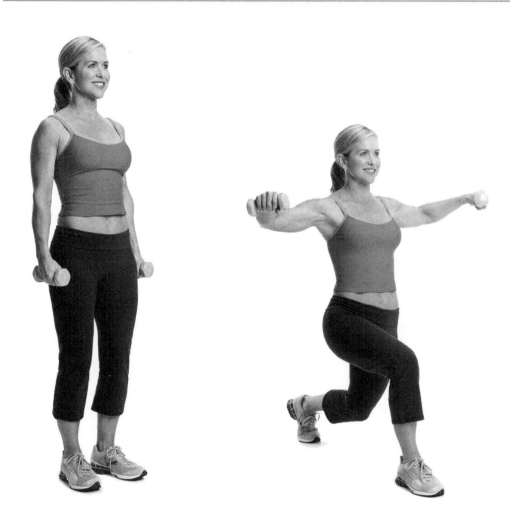

Stand with your feet hip-width apart, holding weights down by your sides, palms facing in.

Take a giant step back with your left leg, then bend your knees to lower your hips toward the floor until your right thigh is parallel to the floor. As you lower, simultaneously lift the weights straight out from your sides until both arms are parallel to the floor. Press back up to the starting position, lowering the weights as you come back to a stand. Complete a set, then switch legs.

SKI HOP

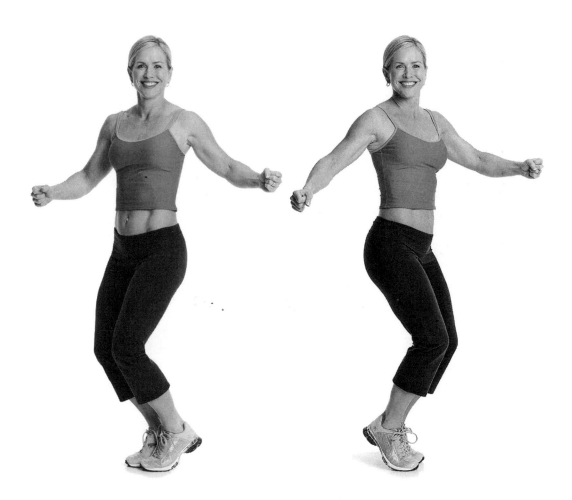

With your feet together, jump from side to side, landing with your knees bent. The wider you jump and the lower you squat into the jump, the harder you'll work. Do this Cardio Quick Take for 1 minute.

BRIDGE "BUN" LIFT

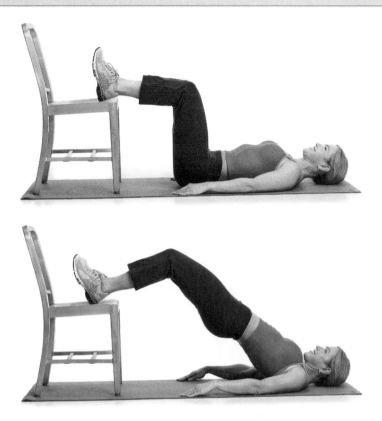

Lie on the floor and place your heels hip-width apart on the edge of a chair seat (or on a step, if a chair is too high), arms down by your sides, palms down.

Keeping your hips square to the ceiling and your navel pulled toward your spine, press into your heels, squeeze your buns, and lift your hips toward the ceiling so your body forms a straight line from your knees to your shoulders. You can use your hands for balance but not to push yourself up. Lower back to the starting position.

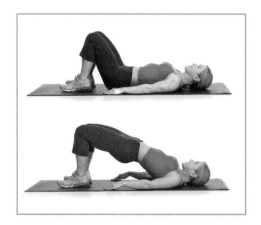

Beginners can try this first without a chair, feet on the floor.

WORKOUT B

Do 12 to 15 repetitions of each of the strength exercises, and do each Cardio Quick Takes exercise for 1 minute. Then repeat the whole workout.

Stair Blaster

Plié

Speed Skating

Stationary Lunge

Squat Hop

STAIR BLASTER

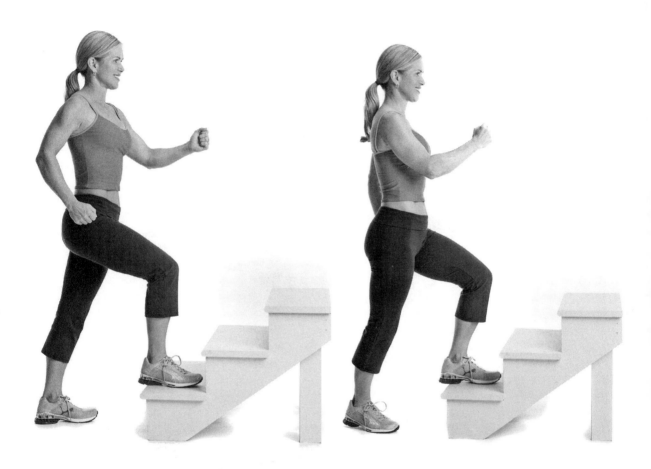

Stand facing a step. Briskly step up with your right and left foot and then down with your right and left foot. Do this Cardio Quick Take for 1 minute.

PLIÉ

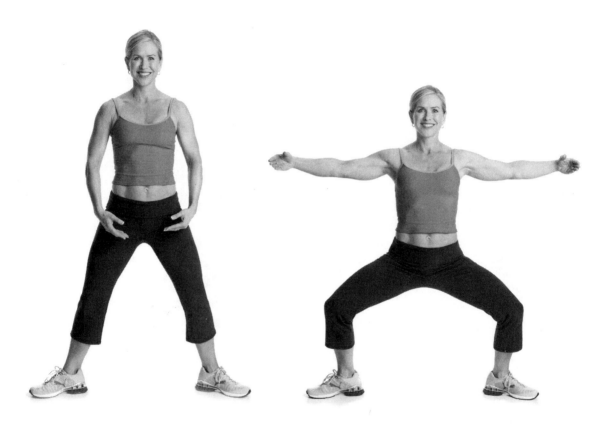

Stand with your feet farther than shoulder-width apart, toes pointing out.

Raise your arms straight out to the sides, palms facing forward. Keeping your back straight, extend your knees over your toes and tuck your tailbone underneath you as if you were sliding down an imaginary wall. Then press into your feet and squeeze your buns to rise back to the starting position.

For a more advanced exercise, deepen your range of motion, trying to get your thighs parallel to the floor.

SPEED SKATING

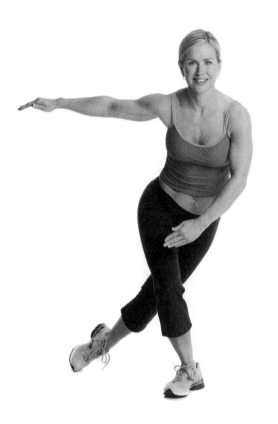 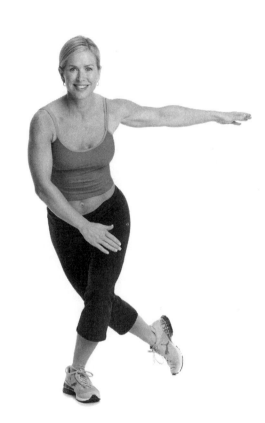

Starting with your feet together, bend your knees and, with your right leg, jump to your right, keeping your body low and landing with a bent right knee. Immediately sweep your left foot behind your right ankle, push off, and jump to your left. Do this Cardio Quick Take for 1 minute.

STATIONARY LUNGE

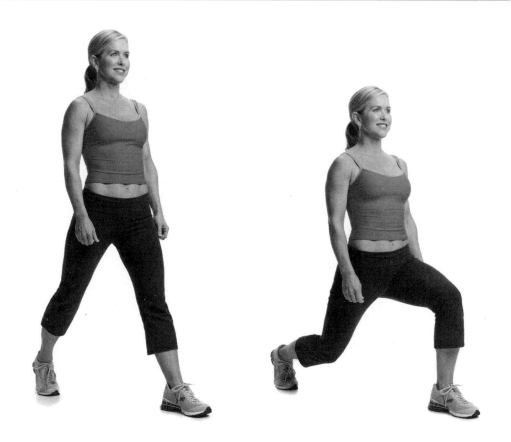

Stand in a split stance: front foot flat on the floor, back heel raised.

Bend both knees and lower into a lunge, keeping your front knee directly above the ankle and your back knee pointing down at the floor. Keep your abs tight, chest lifted, and spine long. Lower your body only as far as is comfortable. Don't bend your knees more than 90 degrees. Squeeze through your buns to raise yourself back up.

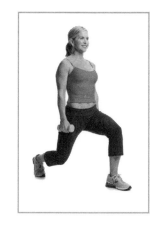

For a more advanced exercise, hold hand weights. Do a full set, then switch legs.

SQUAT HOP

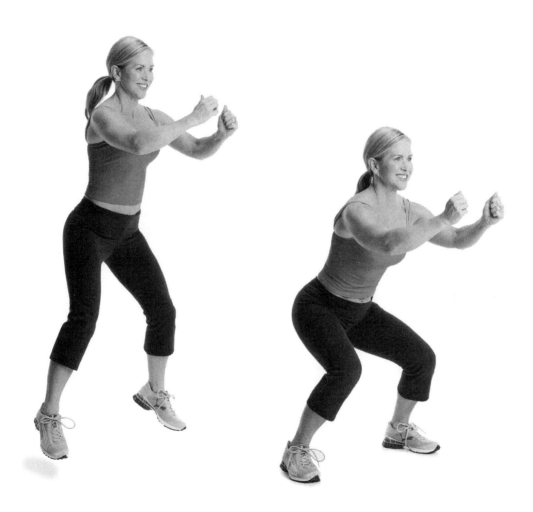

Stand with your feet wide. Lower into a squat and hop forward four times, keeping your feet wide and your legs bent into a squat. Walk back and repeat. Do this Cardio Quick Take for 1 minute.

WORKOUT C

Do 12 to 15 repetitions of each of the strength exercises, and do each Cardio Quick Takes exercise for 1 minute. Then repeat the whole workout.

Curtsy Lunge

Basketball Jump Shot

Simple Squat

Squat/Overhead Press

Tire Drill

CURTSY LUNGE

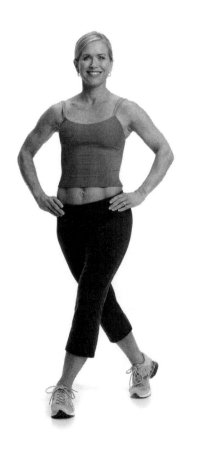
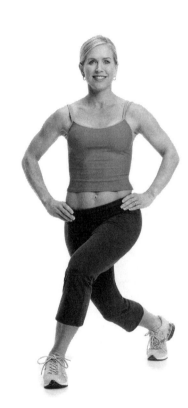

Stand with your feet hip-width apart, hands on your hips. With your right leg, take a giant step back and to the left so that if you were standing on a clock facing 12, your right foot would end up at the 8 o'clock position.

Keeping your back straight and your head up, bend your knees to lower your hips toward the floor until your left thigh is parallel to the ground. Press into your left leg to rise back to the starting position. Complete a full set, then switch sides.

BASKETBALL JUMP SHOT

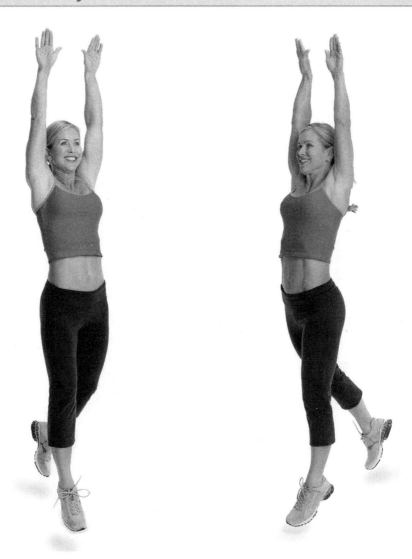

Pretend to shoot some hoops. Step forward on one foot and hop up into the air as if to dunk a basketball. Alternate feet, stepping and hopping. You can step up onto a step to add intensity. Do this Cardio Quick Take for 1 minute.

SIMPLE SQUAT

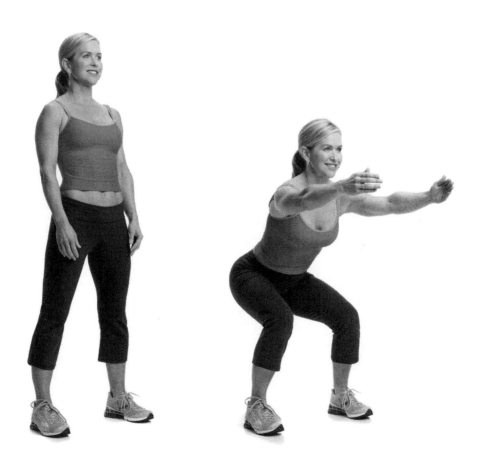

Stand with your feet hip-width apart, toes facing forward, abs tight, and arms at your sides.

Bend your knees to lower your body into a squat position, going as low as you can but no farther than knees bent to 90 degrees. Pretend you are sitting back into a chair—stick out your buns, keep your chest lifted and spine long, and extend your arms out in front of you—and keep your knees above your ankles. Push through your heels and squeeze your buns to rise back to the starting position.

SQUAT/OVERHEAD PRESS

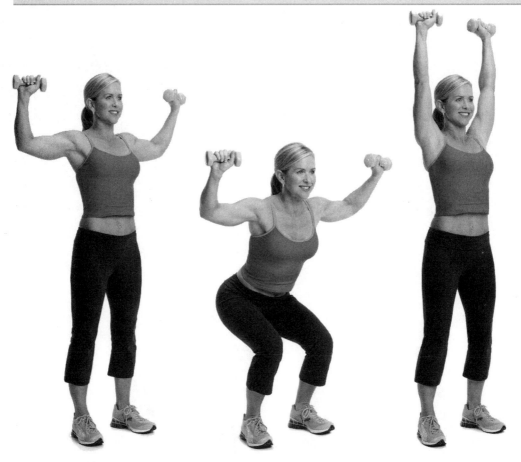

Stand tall with your feet hip-width apart, holding weights in both hands. Begin with your arms bent in the goalpost position: at 90-degree angles out to the sides, with straight wrists and tight abs.

Bend your knees to lower your body into a squat position, going as low as you can but no farther than knees bent to 90 degrees. Pretend you are sitting back into a chair—stick out your buns, keep your chest lifted and spine long, and extend your arms out in front of you—and keep your knees above your ankles.

Push through your heels and squeeze your buns to rise back up. As you reach a standing position, immediately extend your arms to press the weights overhead. Lower them back to the goalpost position.

TIRE DRILL

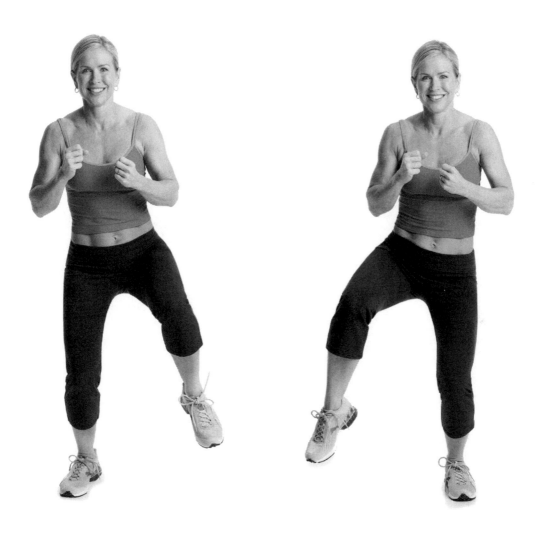

Standing with your feet wide apart and your knees bent about 45 degrees, lift one knee and then the other, taking short quick steps forward as though you were running through tires. Do this Cardio Quick Take for 1 minute.

BEAUTIFUL BOOTY LOG

Make photocopies of this log and use them to keep track of each and every one of the *Prevention's* Shortcuts you take. Three to 5 days a week, you want to check off at least one Beautiful Booty workout. Check off one of the cardio walking workouts every day, and do a second one at least 3 days a week. Also remember to give yourself extra credit every time you squeeze in a 1-Minute Wonder, Lifestyle Shortcut, or *Prevention's* Shortcut from other chapters.

	SUN	MON	TUES	WED	THU	FRI	SAT
Beautiful Booty							
Workout A							
Workout B							
Workout C							
Cardio (see Chapter 4)							
Need for Speed							
Fast and Focused							
Strong and Steady							
Pyramid Power							
Rolling Hills							
Conquer the Mountain							
1-Minute Wonder							
Let Your Feet Do the Walking (page 36)							
Tap Your Toes! (page 76)							
Do "Invisible" Exercise (page 99)							
Multitasking Moves (page 149)							
Stealth Leg Slimmers (page 243)							
Sneaky Arm Shapers (page 295)							

	SUN	MON	TUES	WED	THU	FRI	SAT
Armchair Athletics (page 328)							
Lifestyle Shortcut							
Walk This Way (page 77)							
Take It Outside! (page 80)							
Take Action! (page 144)							
Just Say No (page 178)							
Use Flower Power (page 179)							
Think Positive! (page 180)							
Get Sleep! (page 190)							
Drink Up! (page 191)							
Laugh It Up . . . and Off (page 297)							
Hit the Pound (page 299)							
Hoop It Up (page 329)							
Step Up to the Plate (page 358)							
Live for the Future (page 360)							
Other *Prevention*'s Shortcuts							

Notes (goals, feelings, etc.): _____

_____

_____

_____

_____

_____

_____

_____

EAT YOUR ANTIOXIDANTS

When you're pushing those powerful lower body muscles, it's natural to feel a little postexercise muscle soreness. Cooling down and stretching after a hard workout can help keep some tenderness at bay, as can a healthy diet that includes plenty of antioxidants.

Oxygen, an essential element for life, can create cell-damaging molecules called free radicals during normal cellular metabolism. Research shows free radicals may contribute to everything from cancer and heart disease to wrinkles and, you guessed it, muscle soreness. Antioxidants help quell free radicals and their ill effects by binding to free radicals and transforming them into nondamaging compounds and helping to repair cellular damage. Some of the most well-researched antioxidants include vitamin C, vitamin E, the carotenoids (like beta-carotene), and selenium.

MORE REASONS TO KEEP YOUR REAR IN GEAR

Want to hear a scary statistic? As our bums get bigger, doctors need bigger needles to inoculate us. In a study of 50 men and women who received shots in the butt, 68 percent didn't get the full dose because the medicine got trapped in fat. Medicine must reach muscle to work. If it gets stuck in fat, you could end up with an infection on top of being sick. Okay, that's gross. But it's true! Here are some other incentives for shrinking your posterior.

- You'll be more comfortable in those tiny airplane seats.

- More blue jeans will fit you off the rack.

- It's easier to snuggle with your family on the love seat.

- Bike seats will feel more comfortable—that's the truth. People think that fat back there will provide a "cushion." But the fact is, thick, firm muscle tissue prevents the seat from pressing hard against your sitting bones.

- Family vacation pictures will be more flattering.

- Walking up and down the stairs will feel almost effortless.

- You'll smile when you shop for swimsuits.

Scientists are discovering new antioxidants all the time, many in places we never expected, like your morning cup of coffee. But by far the best sources for these cellular superstars are fruits and vegetables.

The highest concentrations of antioxidants are found in the most deeply or brightly colored fruits and vegetables like spinach, broccoli, cantaloupes, sweet potatoes, apricots, carrots, red bell peppers, and tomatoes. For more vitamin E, include more wheat germ, nuts, seeds, and whole grains in your diet. Selenium can be found in a variety of foods, including fish, shellfish, red meat, grains, eggs, chicken, and garlic.

COMPLEMENT, DON'T COVER UP

Humorist Dave Barry once joked that while men could have moss growing on their butts and barely care or notice, somewhere "between 110 and 115 percent" of all women are extremely vigilant about not exposing theirs, no matter what they look like. "They never emerge from the water [at the beach] without instantly transforming into Buttocks Concealment Mode," he once wrote—which is so funny because it's so true. What's not funny, however, is that I've seen women actually avoid exercise situations because they're so self-conscious about their lower half. Fortunately, most of the *Prevention*'s Shortcuts exercises can be done in the privacy of your own home (though swimming, biking, hiking, and walking will all speed up the results).

This is not a fashion book, of course. But if being more comfortable with how you look from behind helps you make forward progress, I'm all for it. So I consulted with some of my friends in the styling business for advice on flattering your figure while you're firming up. Here are some of my favorite tips.

Go monochrome. Celebrities and stylish New Yorkers deck themselves out in black for a reason—dark colors are indeed slimming. Choose black or dark, muted shades, especially for your lower half. If you love color, add a splash on your torso for a balanced, stylish look.

Add a little flare. Traditional workout tights that hug the ankles draw attention to the shape of your hips and butt. That's why so many women throw XL T-shirts over them. Here's a better approach. Buy a pair of boot-cut or flared workout pants. These pants are loose from the knee or thigh down, flaring out around the ankle to add a point of interest lower on the leg and make your body look balanced.

Skim your hips. Forget the baggy, shapeless Ts. They only draw attention to what you're trying to hide. Instead, pick a shirt that has a more tailored fit and skims right at your hips. By wearing something slightly smaller that gives your body a little shape and form, you actually look about 10 pounds slimmer than when you wear oversize clothes.

Picking a thigh-high swimsuit can be particularly troublesome for women who are large in the lower half. But the right suit can provide coverage while also creating a slimming illusion. Choose one with a diagonal cut at the thigh, because that plays down the buns. As recommended earlier, go with the darker hues.

CHAPTER 11

Sexy, Sleeveless Arms

I knew weight training had finally become mainstream when I saw a feature on "wedding dress workout" arm exercises in a bridal magazine. The feature recommended doing biceps curls, bench dips, and overhead presses (all moves you'll find in the *Prevention*'s Shortcuts plan) to get your arms and shoulders ready to show off in a halter, strapless, or spaghetti-strap dress on your big day. Since then, I've fielded hundreds of questions each year from women who want to know how to shape their shoulders and get rid of upper arm flab, so they can wear something besides long sleeves.

Strong arms are also a great confidence builder for women. A woman with shapely, defined arms looks (and feels) like she can take care of herself. And since many women are bottom heavy to begin with, sculpting the shoulders, biceps, and triceps creates visual balance to the body, making everything look better. As one woman I know enthused after a few months of successful upper body work, "When you've got great arms, everything else falls in line!"

Why do so many women find their arms "unbareable" to begin with? Because like our hips and thighs, the back of the upper arm is a spot where women typically store fat. (When you get your body fat tested with calipers, you'll note they test that spot.) Without healthy diet and exercise, that fat storage combined with flabby triceps muscles can leave you with the jiggly appearance most women hate. The good news is that upper-arm work provides quick gratification. Women often lose weight in their upper body first—in one Penn State study, women exercisers dropped a whopping 31 percent of their arm fat in just 6 months. And since you have proportionately less fat there to begin with, you see results sooner.

Beyond looking good, being stronger is empowering. I guarantee you'll also get a kick out of how much stronger and self-reliant these upper body exercises will make you. Instead of immediately handing over stubborn jars for your husband to open for you, you'll be twisting them off with ease. Garbage bags and laundry baskets will suddenly feel lighter. My girlfriend and I laugh that with our strong arms, we are free to completely rearrange the family room furniture all by ourselves! Together, the two of us move armoires, couches, tables—you name it—whenever we want to give our living spaces a brand new look!

Research shows that women, in particular, are motivated by the functional benefits of strength training. In a study of 44 men and women who lifted weights for 3 months, researchers asked the volunteers what made them feel better about their bodies. Men immediately pointed to looser pants and a better reflection in the mirror. Women liked that, too, but got an even bigger boost from being stronger and better able to lift heavier stuff.

The *Prevention's* Shortcuts arm workouts are designed to incorporate all the muscles in your shoulders (front, middle, and back) as well as your biceps (the front of your upper arm) and triceps (back of upper arm) for a balanced, beautiful appearance. Performing the pushing, pulling, and rowing moves will give you firm, shapely shoulders and arms that you'll love to show off in short sleeves. These moves will also help you stand taller, with a strong midback, improving your posture. When you stand taller, you look slimmer and have more confidence!

Start today, and your arms will look sleeker and stronger in just 4 to 6 weeks. Do one workout from this chapter 3 to 5 days a week. If you feel highly motivated or have extra time, you can do more than one workout in a day, but that's not necessary. I've provided three different arm workouts—A, B, and C—and you can choose whichever one(s) you like, though I recommend mixing them up rather than doing the same one every time. I also recommend plenty of cardio—at least one of the Chapter 4 workouts every day, plus a second one of those workouts 3 to 5 days a week. And whenever possible, try a Lifestyle Shortcut, a 1-Minute Wonder, or any of the *Prevention's* Shortcuts workouts from any other chapters in the book that strike you as fun and interesting. Use the log on page 293 to keep track of what you've done each day.

WORKOUT A

For each exercise, do three sets of 12 to 15 repetitions. You can either do all three sets of a single exercise consecutively or do one set of every exercise (which should take just a bit more than 3 minutes!) and then repeat two more times. Keep your shoulders down and relaxed throughout these moves to avoid straining your muscles or neck and wasting energy.

Pushup

Overhead Shoulder Press

Lateral Raise

Double-Arm Row

Triceps Overhead Press

PUSHUP

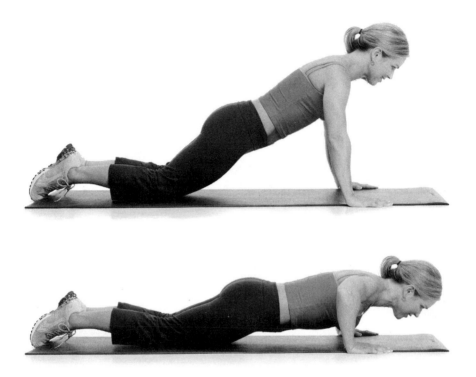

Stretch out on the mat, facedown, in plank position with your arms straight and your hands flat on the floor, a little farther than shoulder-width apart. If you are a beginner, start with your knees on the floor.

Keeping your core tight and level, bend your elbows to 90 degrees to lower your body, keeping your abs tight. Don't sag in the middle. Push back up to the starting position.

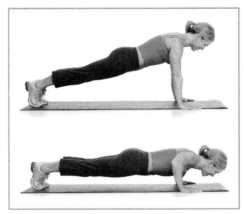

If you are more advanced, rest your toes on the floor, rather than your knees. This takes more core body strength.

OVERHEAD SHOULDER PRESS

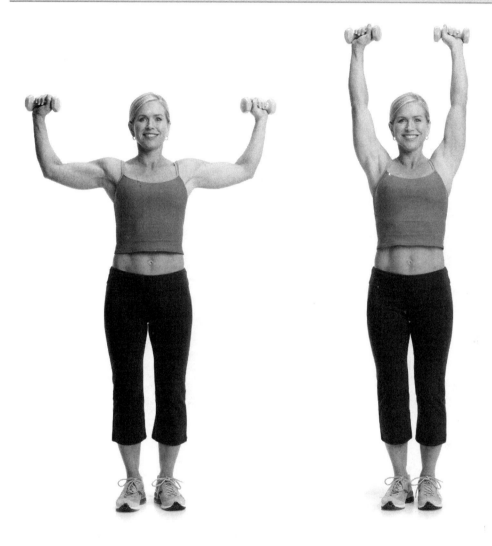

Stand tall with your feet shoulder-width apart, holding weights in both hands. Begin with your arms bent in the goalpost position: at 90-degree angles out to the sides, with straight wrists and tight abs.

Lift your arms overhead until they are straight. Lower back to the starting position.

LATERAL RAISE

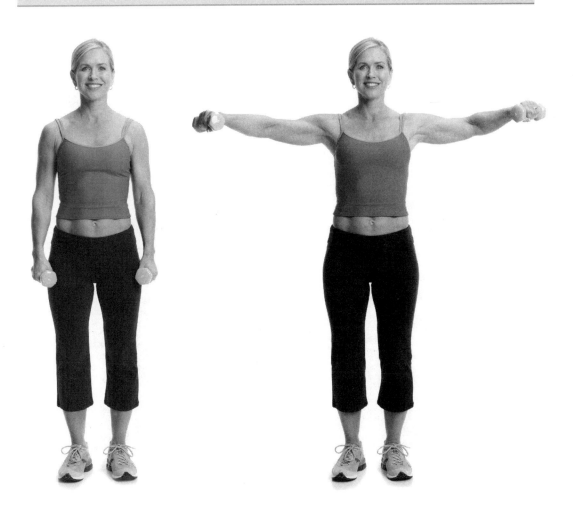

Standing with your feet hip-width apart, hold weights at your sides, palms facing each other.

Keeping your elbows slightly bent, raise your arms straight out to the sides until they are parallel to the floor. Do not raise your arms above shoulder level. Keep your shoulders relaxed—don't shrug! Lower back to the starting position.

DOUBLE-ARM ROW

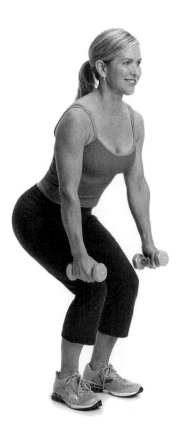
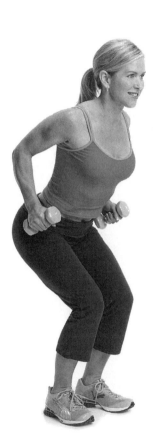

Standing with your feet hip- to shoulder-width apart, knees slightly bent, hold a weight in each hand. Leaning slightly forward from the hips, squat down toward an imaginary chair, keeping your back flat and abs tight. Allow your arms to hang down toward the floor, palms facing in.

Pull your elbows back like you're rowing a boat and squeeze your shoulder blades together to lift the weights to either side of your ribs. Lower back to the starting position.

TRICEPS OVERHEAD PRESS

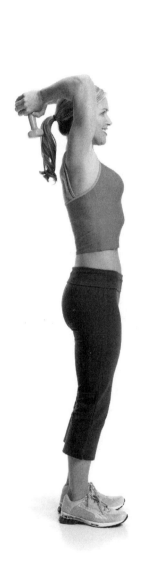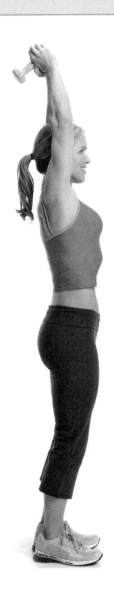

Stand with your feet hip-width apart (or sit in a chair). Clasp one weight with both hands. Extend your arms straight overhead, elbows close to your ears.

Bend your elbows to slowly lower the weight behind you. Keep your elbows close to your ears. Contract your triceps and straighten your elbows to return to the starting position.

WORKOUT B

For each exercise, do three sets of 12 to 15 repetitions. You can either do all three sets of a single exercise consecutively or do one set of every exercise (which should take just a bit more than 3 minutes!) and then repeat two more times. Keep your shoulders down and relaxed throughout these moves to avoid straining your muscles or neck and wasting energy.

Front Shoulder Raise

Reverse Fly

Biceps Curl

Triceps Overhead Press

Chest Fly

FRONT SHOULDER RAISE

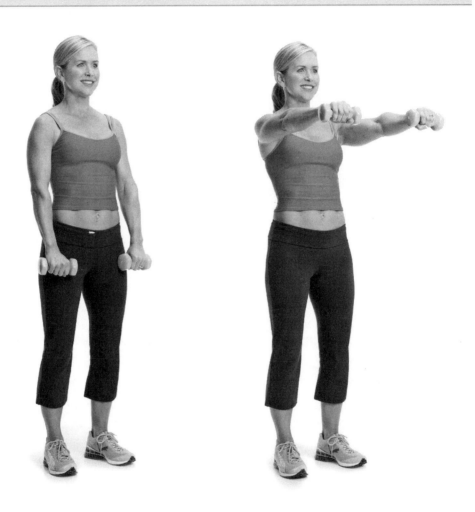

Standing with your feet hip-width apart, hold weights down in front of your thighs, palms facing you.

Keeping your elbows slightly bent, raise your arms straight up in front of you until they are parallel to the floor. Keep your shoulders relaxed—don't shrug! Do not raise your arms above shoulder level. Lower back to the starting position.

REVERSE FLY

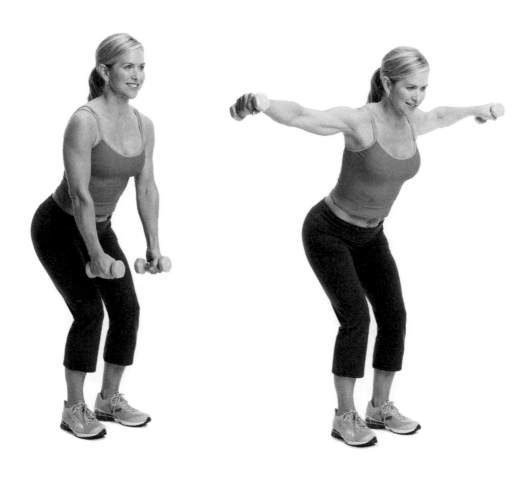

Standing with your feet hip- to shoulder-width apart, knees slightly bent, hold a weight in each hand. Lean slightly forward from the hips, keeping your back flat and abs tight. Allow your arms to hang toward the floor, palms facing each other.

Squeeze your shoulder blades together as you lift the weights, extending your arms out to the sides like airplane wings. Make sure to relax your neck. Don't squeeze or scrunch your shoulders. Lower back to the starting position.

BICEPS CURL

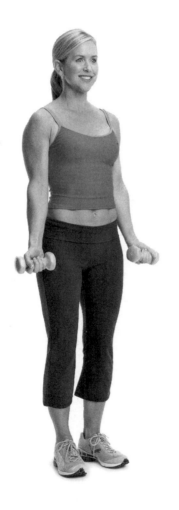 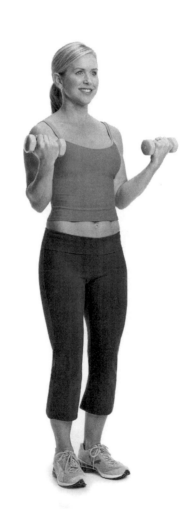

Stand with your feet hip- to shoulder-width apart, knees bent slightly. Hold a weight in each hand with your arms down by your sides, palms facing forward.

Bend your elbows to lift the weights toward your shoulders, stopping when they are at chest height, palms facing your body. Slowly lower back to the starting position.

TRICEPS OVERHEAD PRESS

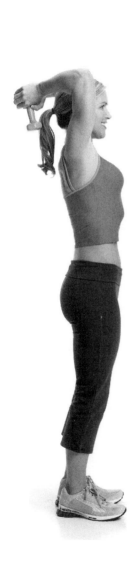 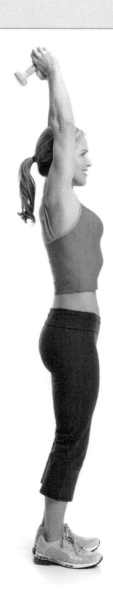

Stand with your feet hip-width apart (or sit in a chair). Clasp one weight with both hands. Extend your arms straight overhead, elbows close to your ears.

Bend your elbows to slowly lower the weight behind you. Keep your elbows close to your ears. Contract your triceps and straighten your elbows to return to the starting position.

CHEST FLY

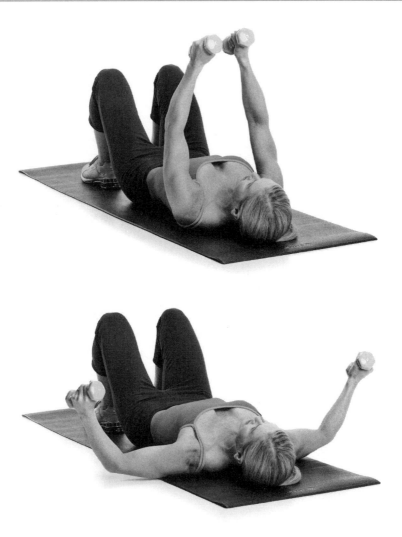

Lie faceup on the floor with your legs bent and your feet flat. Hold weights up over your chest with your arms extended, elbows slightly bent, and palms facing each other.

Slowly open your arms out to the sides, allowing the weights to fall to about the 10 o'clock and 2 o'clock positions. Then slowly lift your arms back to the starting position. Focus on squeezing through your chest as if you were hugging a large tree.

WORKOUT C

For each exercise, do three sets of 12 to 15 repetitions. You can either do all three sets of a single exercise consecutively or do one set of every exercise (which should take just a bit more than 3 minutes!) and then repeat two more times. Keep your shoulders down and relaxed throughout these moves to avoid straining your muscles or neck and wasting energy.

Double-Arm Row

Lateral Shoulder Raise

Overhead Shoulder Press

Pushup

Triceps Dip on Chair

DOUBLE-ARM ROW

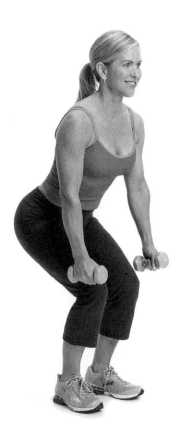
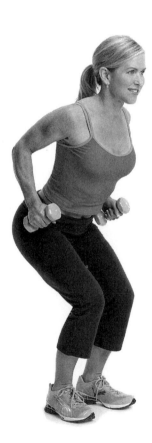

Standing with your feet hip- to shoulder-width apart, knees slightly bent, hold a weight in each hand. Leaning slightly forward from the hips, squat down toward an imaginary chair, keeping your back flat and abs tight. Allow your arms to hang down toward the floor, palms facing in.

Pull your elbows back like you're rowing a boat and squeeze your shoulder blades together to lift the weights to either side of your ribs. Lower back to the starting position.

LATERAL SHOULDER RAISE

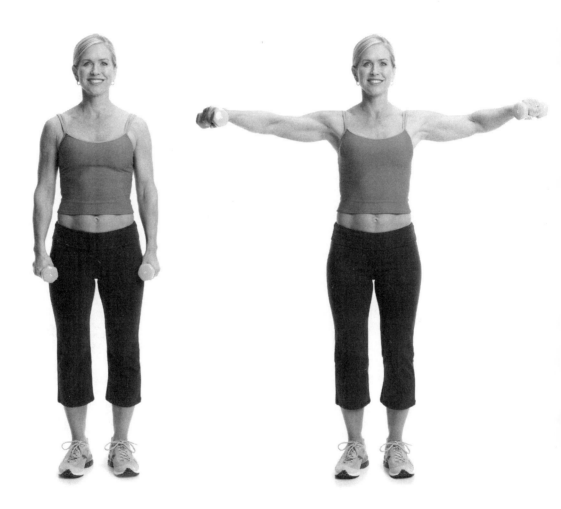

Standing with your feet hip-width apart, hold weights at your sides, palms facing each other.

Keeping your elbows slightly bent, raise your arms straight out to the sides until they are parallel to the floor. Do not raise your arms above shoulder level. Keep your shoulders relaxed—don't shrug! Lower back to the starting position.

OVERHEAD SHOULDER PRESS

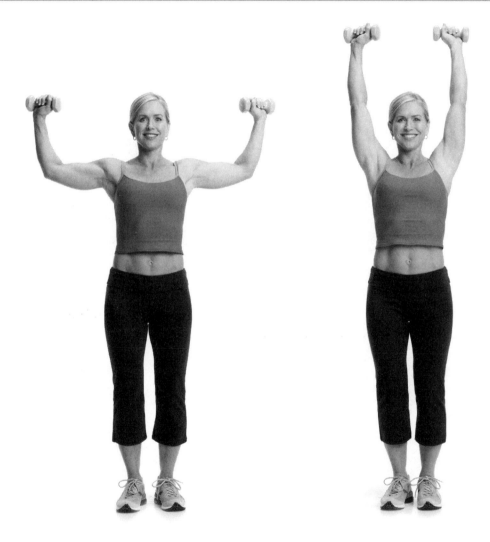

Stand tall with your feet shoulder-width apart, holding weights in both hands. Begin with your arms bent in the goalpost position: at 90-degree angles out to the sides, with straight wrists and tight abs.

Lift your arms overhead until they are straight. Lower back to the starting position.

PUSHUP

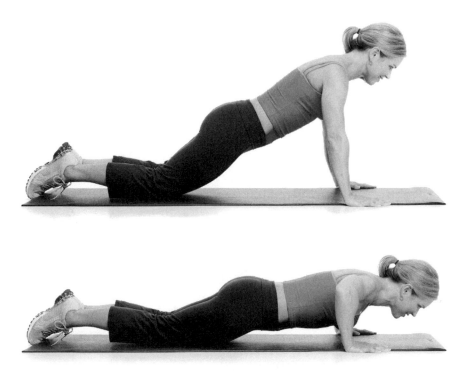

Stretch out on the mat, facedown, in plank position with your arms straight and your hands flat on the floor, a little farther than shoulder-width apart. If you are a beginner, start with your knees on the floor.

Keeping your core tight and level, bend your elbows to 90 degrees to lower your body, keeping your abs tight. Don't sag in the middle. Push back up to the starting position.

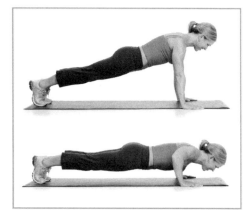

If you are more advanced, rest your toes on the floor, rather than your knees. This takes more core body strength.

TRICEPS DIP ON CHAIR

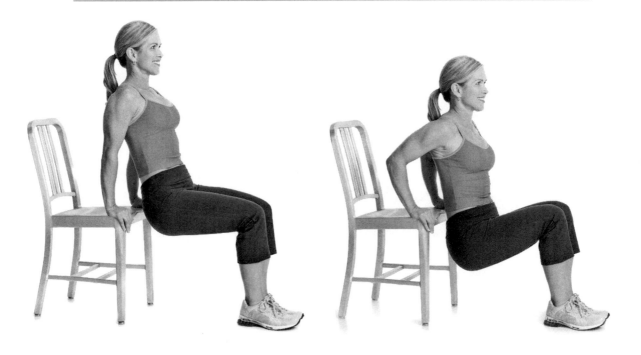

Sit on the edge of a chair, grasping the seat with a hand at either side of your hips. Slide your buns off the seat while walking your feet forward.

Bend your elbows straight back, lowering your hips toward the floor until your elbows are in line with your shoulders. Press back up to the starting position.

Advanced exercisers can straighten one or both legs.

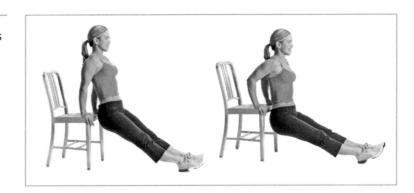

SEXY, SLEEVELESS ARMS LOG

Make photocopies of this log and use them to keep track of each and every one of the *Prevention*'s Shortcuts you take. Three to 5 days a week, you want to check off at least one arm workout. Check off one of the cardio walking workouts every day, and do a second one at least 3 days a week. Also remember to give yourself extra credit every time you squeeze in a 1-Minute Wonder, Lifestyle Shortcut, or *Prevention*'s Shortcut from another chapter.

	SUN	MON	TUES	WED	THU	FRI	SAT
Sexy, Sleeveless Arms							
Workout A							
Workout B							
Workout C							
Cardio (see Chapter 4)							
Need for Speed							
Fast and Focused							
Strong and Steady							
Pyramid Power							
Rolling Hills							
Conquer the Mountain							
1-Minute Wonder							
Let Your Feet Do the Walking (page 36)							
Tap Your Toes! (page 76)							
Do "Invisible" Exercise (page 99)							
Multitasking Moves (page 149)							
Stealth Leg Slimmers (page 243)							
Sneaky Arm Shapers (page 295)							

(continued)

	SUN	MON	TUES	WED	THU	FRI	SAT
Armchair Athletics (page 328)							
Lifestyle Shortcut							
Walk This Way (page 77)							
Take It Outside! (page 80)							
Take Action! (page 144)							
Just Say No (page 178)							
Use Flower Power (page 179)							
Think Positive! (page 180)							
Get Sleep! (page 190)							
Drink Up! (page 191)							
Laugh It Up . . . and Off (page 297)							
Hit the Pound (page 299)							
Hoop It Up (page 329)							
Step Up to the Plate (page 358)							
Live for the Future (page 360)							
Other *Prevention*'s Shortcuts							

Notes (goals, feelings, etc.): _____

_____

_____

_____

_____

_____

_____

WRIST WATCH

Pushups and other pressing exercises are terrific upper body toners, but as they say, you're only as strong as your weakest link—and for many women, that's their wrists. Many women complain that they can't perform pushups or yoga positions like planks because they feel pain in their wrists. A quick way to ease the ache is to hold a light weight in each hand, so the weights run parallel to your body, and perform the moves with your wrists completely straight, rather than bent. You can also perform exercises to strengthen the muscles that support your wrists.

They don't grab the same head-turning attention as shapely shoulders and beautiful biceps, but your forearms are an equally important part of the picture.

1-MINUTE WONDER
SNEAKY ARM SHAPERS

You don't have to wait to do your *Prevention*'s Shortcuts arm routines to tone your arms. There are dozens of opportunities every day to make those muscles stronger and more toned. Here are just a few of my favorites.

Shop and curl. As you shop, pulse your grocery basket up and down, doing mini biceps curls in the shopping aisle. The longer you shop, the more challenging the move becomes!

Baby bounce. If you have a baby or young toddler, lie on your back, holding the child on your chest. Carefully extend your arms and "press" her toward the ceiling—enjoying the view of her giggling while you do—then lower her back down.

Wall push. Pushups can be performed practically anywhere there's a wall or flat surface. Just put your hands on the wall or counter, lean in, and push up. My cowriter does them against the kitchen counter while dinner cooks.

T stretch. Stuck at your desk? Take a break to stretch your arms straight out from your sides, palms down, and extend through your fingertips. Keep your shoulders down and relaxed but active. Hold for 10 to 30 seconds. You'll really feel the effort in your middle shoulder muscles.

Ball squeeze. Keep a tennis ball or some hand putty by your computer, and periodically take squeeze breaks to exercise your hands and work the muscles in your forearms.

Strengthening them will help reduce wrist strain. If you're plagued by wrist pain, add wrist curls to your arm workouts: Hold a weight in each hand, elbows bent at your sides, forearms straight in front of you, palms facing up. Curl your wrists so your knuckles point toward the ceiling. Return to start. Repeat 12 to 15 times.

If you spend long days doing repetitive tasks, you should also take steps to protect your wrists against carpal tunnel syndrome—a painful, progressive condition caused by compression of one of the major nerves in your wrist. Whether you work in data processing, can't take your hands off your BlackBerry, or engage in any other kind of repetitive hand work, orthopedists recommend that you try to keep your wrists in a straight line with your hands and arms whenever possible (excessive bending seems to contribute to the problem). Also take breaks when possible to shake out and stretch your hands to boost circulation.

ROW, ROW, ROW YOUR BOD

Most women who go to the gym make a beeline for the treadmill or elliptical trainer, barely noticing the bank of rowing machines. Besides the fact that you never have to wait in line for a rowing machine (industry surveys show 76 percent fewer people use rowing machines than treadmills), the biggest reason to use them is calorie burn. Just 10 minutes of rowing burns about the same number of calories as running a mile! What's more, rowing builds beautiful back, biceps, and shoulder muscles. Because you push off with your legs with each stroke, your lower body gets into the act, as does your core, making the rowing machine the best total-body cardio workout in the gym.

GO WITH THE GLOW

Once you've sculpted those sexy arms, you'll be ready to show them off in sleeveless shirts and dresses. A little added attention to skin care can make the most of their debut! Here's what dermatologists recommend.

Smooth them with AHAs. If you look at your freshly shaped arms and see tiny white or reddish bumps, you're not alone. Up to 40 percent of adult men and women have keratosis pilaris, a condition where the skin's top layers don't slough off normally, leaving a dead-skin pileup around the hair follicles. Smooth them over with a moisturizer containing AHAs (alpha hydroxy acids), which will help exfoliate the dead skin. If that doesn't work, take a nice hot bath to soften them, then rub the area with a coarse washcloth.

Rub rough elbows. Our elbows have to be tough to withstand all the propping and rubbing they sustain every day. But the skin doesn't have to show it. An in-shower body scrub (like a salt scrub) will make the skin feel less rough. These exfoliating scrubs are also great for your feet. It's like getting a cheap pedicure. My favorite little indulgence is to get whatever new scrub is available from Bath & Body Works. I love to try a new scent each time I go!

Check for damage. Even if your arms haven't seen the sun since 1975, you can still have sun damage if you spent your youth unprotected—or worse, baking with a bottle of baby oil! Keep an eye out for unusual moles or precancerous areas like rough, scaly patches. Get anything suspicious checked by a dermatologist.

Shield them from the sun. Use sunscreen with an SPF of 15 or higher whenever you go out in the sun. Slather it on liberally and reapply about every hour or two.

LIFESTYLE SHORTCUT
LAUGH IT UP . . . AND OFF

Nothing puts life into perspective like a good laugh. Everyone who knows me knows I love to laugh. So I was tickled to read the results of a recent study that found that laughing out loud for 10 to 15 minutes a day (the amount of laughter you'd get from a *really* funny sitcom) can burn up to 40 calories. Not that that's a huge number, but over the course of a year, it could shave more than 4 pounds from someone who usually doesn't crack a smile.

More important, laughter is your best weapon against stress, which can pile on pounds in multiple ways. Brain research shows that laughter overpowers the stress response (which is why so many of us laugh when we're nervous), and it reminds us that most of the nitty-gritty we worry about is not a matter of life and death. So we might as well lighten up!

The challenges of life can feel so heavy that women can literally forget to be silly! Nowadays, I bypass the dramas in the DVD aisle and head straight for the comedy section! The ultimate medicine for me is working out to something that makes me laugh.

CHAPTER 12

Fantabulous Flexibility

Yogis are fond of saying you're only as young as your spine. Obviously, your spine is exactly the same age in years as the rest of your body, but depending on how you take care of it, it can feel decades older . . . or younger. Which brings us to the goal of the *Prevention*'s Shortcuts program for fantabulous (fantastic *and* fabulous!) flexibility: to keep your spine and the rest of your joints in your arms, legs, shoulders, and hips as young as you want to feel.

There are lots of ways to stretch. You can do static stretching like the moves I describe in Chapter 4, where you use your body weight to hold a pose and stretch specific muscles. You can have a partner stretch you by gently taking your arms and legs through a range of motion. You can even get a Thai massage, which incorporates stretching of your joints along with kneading your muscles (feels awesome!). They all work. But by far the best way to increase flexibility is regular yoga practice.

Yoga has been used for thousands of years to increase flexibility. Yet millions of people who could benefit the most are the least likely to try it. Why? Because they're intimidated. Don't be. The yoga poses I've chosen for the *Prevention*'s Shortcuts workouts are simple and gentle. They're meant to be done in a relaxed fashion without pain or strain, and anyone, regardless of their current flexibility (or lack thereof) can do them. The combination of moves are designed to provide you with a balanced stretching session, concentrating especially on common trouble spots in the hamstrings, back, and hips. Believe me, the men (and many of the women) who show up at my 5:30 a.m. yoga classes are not yogis; they're active people looking for a facili-

LIFESTYLE SHORTCUT
HIT THE POUND

I love my dog! He never talks back. He lies there quietly at my feet, emanating love. And he *always* says yes when I want to go for a walk! He's my morning motivator. My dog, my iPod, and a little sunshine, and I'm set to *go*! If you've been thinking about getting a dog, now's the time to do it. A furry friend could help speed your weight loss progress.

A study from the University of Missouri–Columbia found that walking a dog helped people shed more weight than they would with Weight Watchers or other popular diet plans. The researchers found that when overweight volunteers started walking a dog for just 10 to 20 minutes a day, they lost an average of 14 pounds over the course of a year—all without changing their eating habits. The average diet program yields just a 5- to 7-pound loss in the same amount of time. As a bonus, studies show that dogs can help lower stress and improve your sense of well-being—both of which will help accelerate your goals for weight loss and healthy living.

---

tated stretching session. Now they love it. As we age, we quickly realize that stretching can make all the difference in our range of motion!

The following workouts will increase your flexibility in as little as 3 weeks. Do one workout 3 to 5 days a week. If you feel highly motivated or have extra time, you can do more than one workout in a day, but that's not necessary. I've provided three different flexibility workouts—A, B, and C—and you can choose whichever one(s) you like, though I recommend mixing them up rather than doing the same one every time. Also do plenty of cardio—at least one of the Chapter 4 workouts every day, plus a second one of those workouts 3 to 5 days a week. And whenever possible, try a Lifestyle Shortcut, a 1-Minute Wonder, or any of the *Prevention*'s Shortcuts workouts from any other chapters in the book that strike you as fun and interesting. Use the log on page 325 to keep track of what you've done each day.

WORKOUT A

Hold each pose for 30 to 45 seconds (on each side, where appropriate). Do the entire workout twice.

Crescent Lunge

Downward-Facing Dog

Triangle

Cat/Cow

Cobra

Seated Spinal Twist

Child's Pose

CRESCENT LUNGE

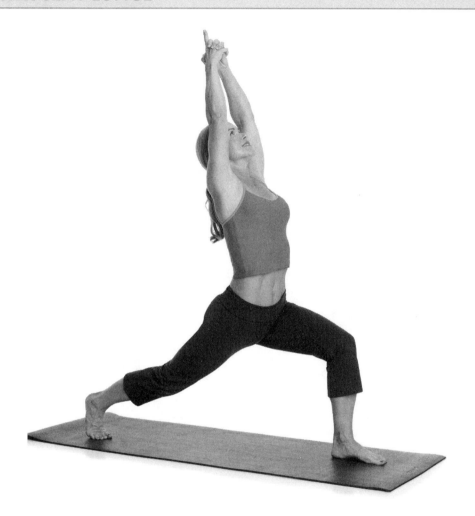

Stand in a lunge position with your right leg forward and bent 90 degrees, your right knee directly over your right ankle. Lower your left knee toward the floor, lifting your breastbone and raising your arms overhead. Clasp your hands together so your index fingers point toward the sky, and look upward, bending backward slightly. Breathe smoothly as you relax into the stretch. Switch sides.

DOWNWARD-FACING DOG

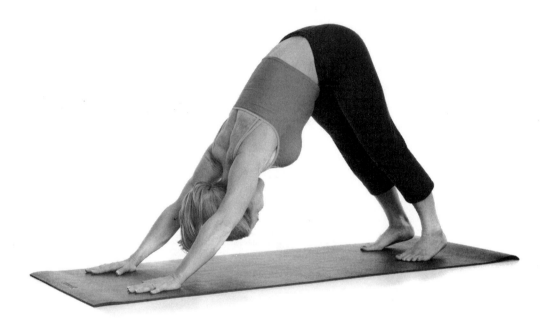

Begin on your hands and knees. Place your feet hip-width apart, toes tucked under. Space your hands shoulder-width apart and press the weight of your body onto your palms, spreading your fingers like starfish. Straighten your legs (beginners can bend their knees) and lift your tailbone toward the sky while pulling your navel toward your spine and gently pushing down through your heels. (Feel the stretch through the backs of your legs.) Open your upper back by rotating your shoulder blades slightly outward. Keep your shoulders away from your ears and relax your head between your arms.

TRIANGLE

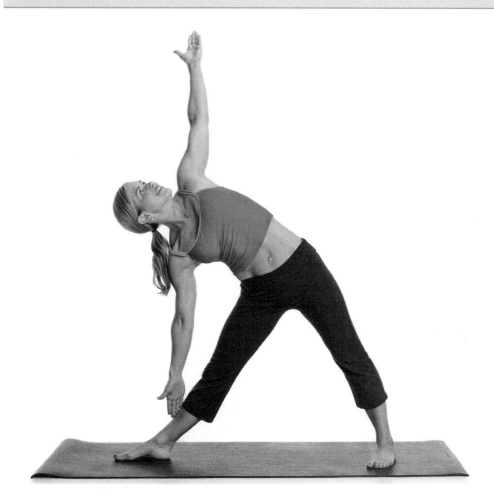

From a standing position, step to the side with your right foot approximately 3 feet from your left. Point your right toes 90 degrees to the right. Move the toes of your left foot slightly to the right so that the foot is gently angled inward. Extend your arms straight out, parallel to the floor, shoulder blades relaxed. Imagine your body is pressed against a pane of glass. Keep your hips stacked on top of each other as you tip over to the right, extending your left arm to the sky. Rest your right arm as far down your right leg as is comfortable. Keep your chest open and look toward the sky. (If this hurts your neck, turn your head toward the floor.) Then switch sides.

CAT/COW

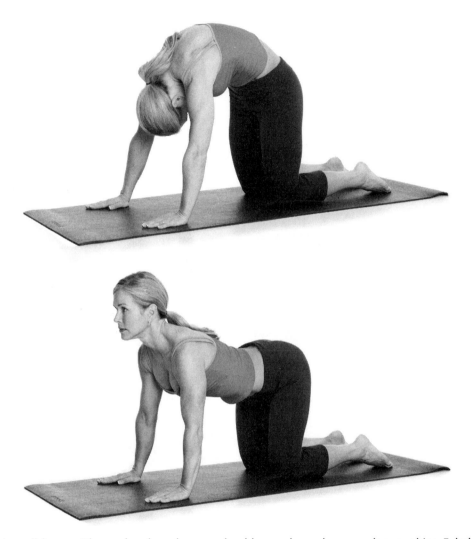

Kneel on all fours, with your hands under your shoulders and your knees under your hips. Exhale and tuck your tailbone under, round your spine, and drop your head as though you are looking for your navel. Push evenly through your hands and knees, and arch your upper back toward the sky.

Continue from Cat into Cow (back extension): Extend your spine, lift your tailbone toward the sky, and drop your belly down toward the floor. Look up. Try to lengthen the crown of your head away from your tailbone.

COBRA

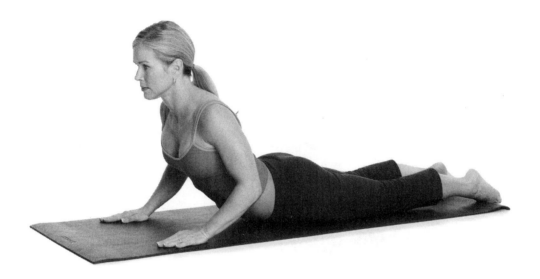

Lie facedown on the floor with your legs extended and the tops of your feet on the floor. Place your hands on the floor beneath your shoulders, hugging your elbows close to your torso. Press your feet, thighs, and pelvis firmly against the floor. Straighten your arms to lift your chest off the floor, raising only as high as comfortably possible, while keeping your hips in contact with the floor. Keep your shoulders down and back, lifting through your breastbone, opening your chest, and extending your spine.

SEATED SPINAL TWIST

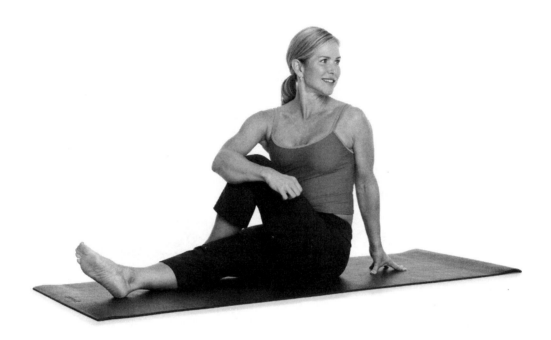

Sit on the floor with your legs extended. Place your hands on the floor behind your back for support. Cross your left leg over the right and place your left foot on the floor on the outside of your right knee. Keeping your spine long and tall, twist your torso toward the left, wrapping your right arm around your left knee. Look over your left shoulder. Hold. Then switch sides.

CHILD'S POSE

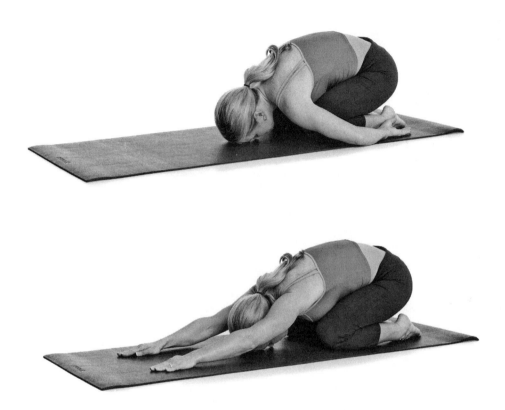

Kneel and then sit with your hips back on your heels. Lower your upper body down over your lap and rest your forehead on the floor. Rest your arms at your sides, palms facing up.

Or you can extend your arms straight out in front of you, reaching and spreading your fingers. Relax your neck, face, and shoulders as you take deep, slow breaths.

WORKOUT B

Hold each pose for 30 to 45 seconds (on each side, where appropriate). Do the entire workout twice.

Chair Pose

Triangle

Pigeon

Downward-Facing Dog

Spinal Balance and Crunch

Cat/Cow

Child's Pose

CHAIR POSE

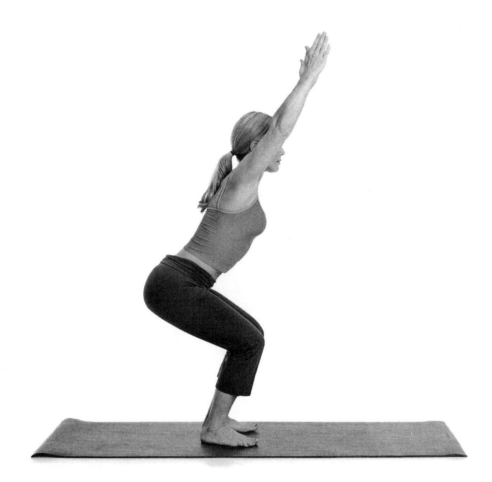

Stand tall, with your feet close together. Raise your arms overhead so they are parallel with each other, palms facing in. Sit in an imaginary chair by bending your knees, trying to lower your thighs as close to parallel to the floor as is comfortably possible. Your knees will project over your feet, and your torso will lean slightly forward, forming a 90-degree angle with the tops of your thighs. Keep your shoulders down and back. Tuck your tailbone forward to lengthen your spine. Hold, and then lift through your arms to release the pose.

TRIANGLE

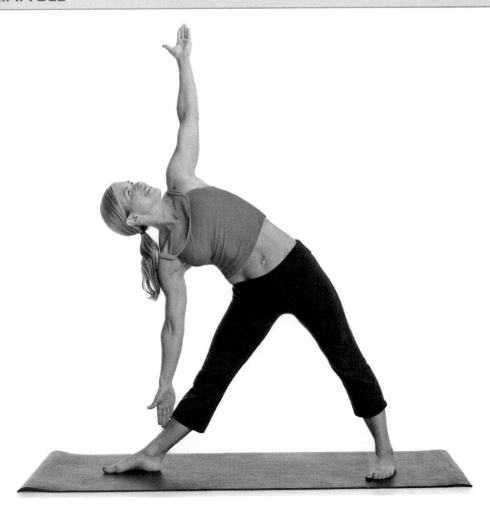

From a standing position, step to the side with your right foot approximately 3 feet from your left. Point your right toes 90 degrees to the right. Move the toes of your left foot slightly to the right so that the foot is gently angled inward. Extend your arms straight out, parallel to the floor, shoulder blades relaxed. Imagine your body is pressed against a pane of glass. Keep your hips stacked on top of each other as you tip over to the right, extending your left arm to the sky. Rest your right arm as far down your right leg as is comfortable. Keep your chest open and look toward the sky. (If this hurts your neck, turn your head toward the floor.) Then switch sides.

PIGEON

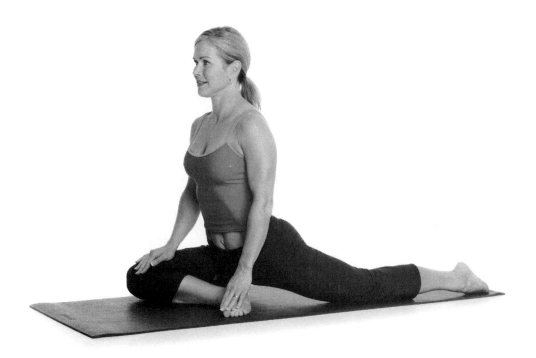

Kneel and then sit with your hips back on your heels. Lift your hips slightly and, keeping your right knee bent, stretch your left leg back to a half-split position. (You can rest your right thigh on the floor so your right foot is positioned in front of your left hip.) Place your left knee on the floor with the leg fully extended. Open your chest and lift your head to look toward the ceiling. Then release and switch legs.

DOWNWARD-FACING DOG

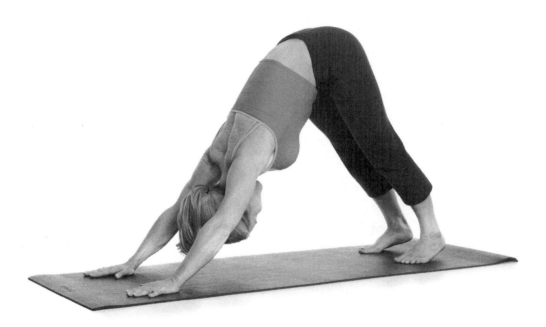

Begin on your hands and knees. Place your feet hip-width apart, toes tucked under. Space your hands shoulder-width apart and press the weight of your body onto your palms, spreading your fingers like starfish. Straighten your legs (beginners can bend their knees) and lift your tailbone toward the sky while pulling your navel toward your spine and gently pushing down through your heels. (Feel the stretch through the backs of your legs.) Open your upper back by rotating your shoulder blades slightly outward. Keep your shoulders away from your ears and relax your head between your arms.

SPINAL BALANCE AND CRUNCH

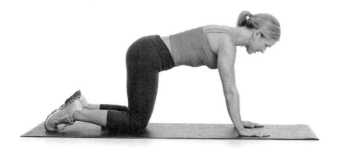

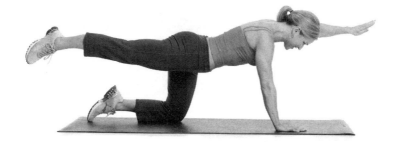

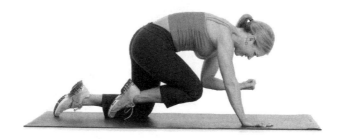

Kneel on all fours, with your hands directly beneath your shoulders and your knees directly beneath your hips. Keep your back straight and your head in line with your spine.

Draw your navel toward your spine and simultaneously raise your left arm and right leg, extending them in line with your back so your fingers are pointing straight ahead and your toes are pointing back. Hold for 2 seconds.

Then contract your abs and draw your left elbow and your right knee together, beneath your torso. Complete a full set, then switch sides.

CAT/COW

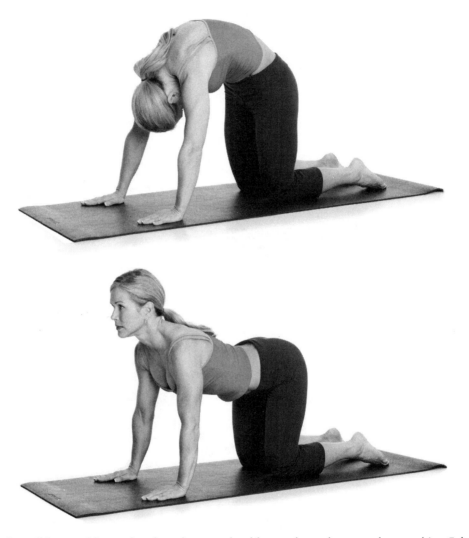

Kneel on all fours, with your hands under your shoulders and your knees under your hips. Exhale and tuck your tailbone under, round your spine, and drop your head as though you are looking for your navel. Push evenly through your hands and knees, and arch your upper back toward the sky.

Continue from Cat into Cow (back extension): Extend your spine, lift your tailbone toward the sky, and drop your belly down toward the floor. Look up. Try to lengthen the crown of your head away from your tailbone.

CHILD'S POSE

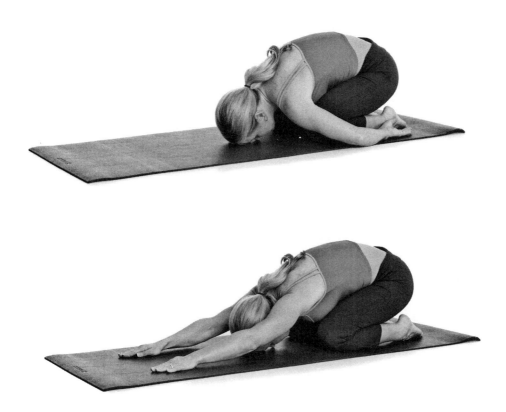

Kneel and then sit with your hips back on your heels. Lower your upper body down over your lap and rest your forehead on the floor. Rest your arms at your sides, palms facing up.

Or you can extend your arms straight out in front of you, reaching and spreading your fingers. Relax your neck, face, and shoulders as you take deep, slow breaths.

WORKOUT C

Hold each pose for 30 to 45 seconds (on each side, where appropriate). Do the entire workout twice.

Downward-Facing Dog

Crescent Lunge

Chair Pose

Seated Butterfly

Half Roll-Back

Seated Spinal Twist

Pigeon

Child's Pose

DOWNWARD-FACING DOG

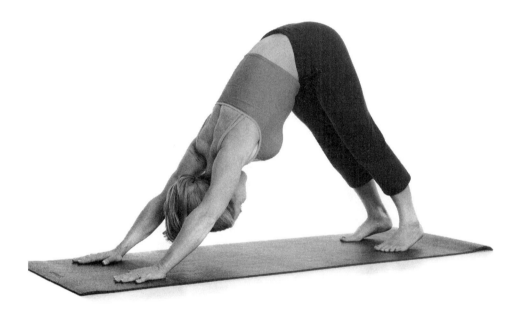

Begin on your hands and knees. Place your feet hip-width apart, toes tucked under. Space your hands shoulder-width apart and press the weight of your body onto your palms, spreading your fingers like starfish. Straighten your legs (beginners can bend their knees) and lift your tailbone toward the sky while pulling your navel toward your spine and gently pushing down through your heels. (Feel the stretch through the backs of your legs.) Open your upper back by rotating your shoulder blades slightly outward. Keep your shoulders away from your ears and relax your head between your arms.

CRESCENT LUNGE

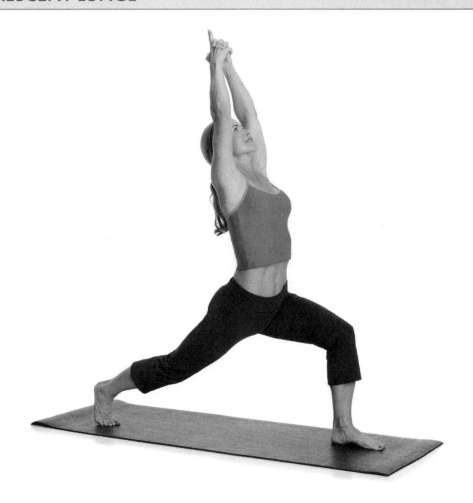

Stand in a lunge position with your right leg forward and bent 90 degrees, your right knee directly over your right ankle. Lower your left knee toward the floor, lifting your breastbone and raising your arms overhead. Clasp your hands together so your index fingers point toward the sky, and look upward, bending backward slightly. Breathe smoothly as you relax into the stretch. Switch sides.

CHAIR POSE

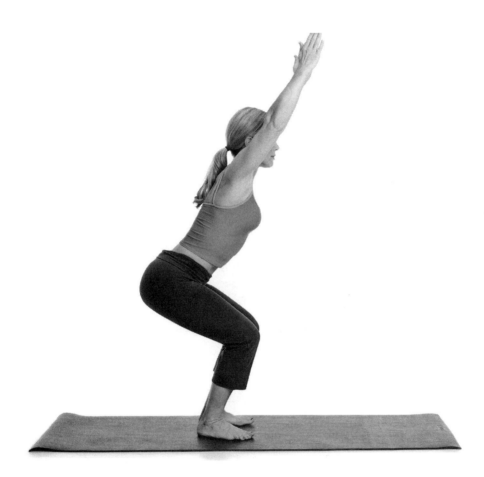

Stand tall, with your feet close together. Raise your arms overhead so they are parallel with each other, palms facing in. Sit in an imaginary chair by bending your knees, trying to lower your thighs as close to parallel to the floor as is comfortably possible. Your knees will project over your feet, and your torso will lean slightly forward, forming a 90-degree angle with the tops of your thighs. Keep your shoulders down and back. Tuck your tailbone forward to lengthen your spine. Hold, and then lift through your arms to release the pose.

SEATED BUTTERFLY

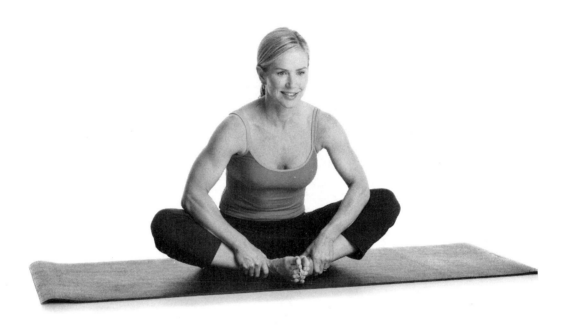

Begin in a seated position with the soles of your feet together. Place your hands on your ankles and press your elbows into your inner thighs. Gently push your knees toward the floor. Press your sitting bones down against the floor and lengthen your spine, reaching toward the sky with the crown of your head. Drop your shoulders away from your ears and gently tuck in your chin. Inhale and exhale a little farther into the stretch.

HALF ROLL-BACK

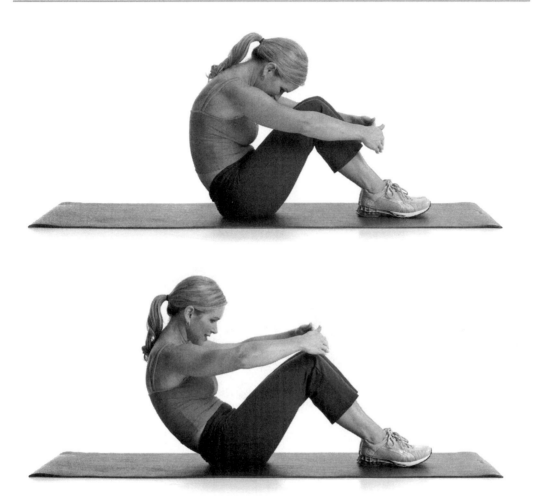

Sit on the floor with your knees bent and your feet and knees separated slightly. Pull your navel toward your spine and curl your spine forward so your torso is bent over your legs in a C shape. Reach your arms forward, with your shoulders relaxed.

Exhale and, maintaining a C shape with your spine, roll halfway back by tucking your tailbone and lowering vertebrae by vertebrae. Inhale and pull your abs even closer toward your spine. Then exhale and contract your abs to return to the starting position. Maintain a rounded spine throughout the movement.

SEATED SPINAL TWIST

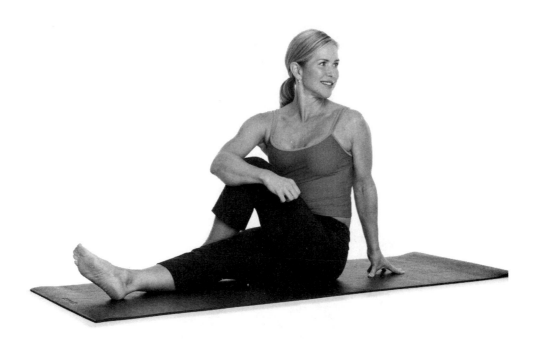

Sit on the floor with your legs extended. Place your hands on the floor behind your back for support. Cross your left leg over the right and place your left foot on the floor on the outside of your right knee. Keeping your spine long and tall, twist your torso toward the left, wrapping your right arm around your left knee. Look over your left shoulder. Hold. Then switch sides.

PIGEON

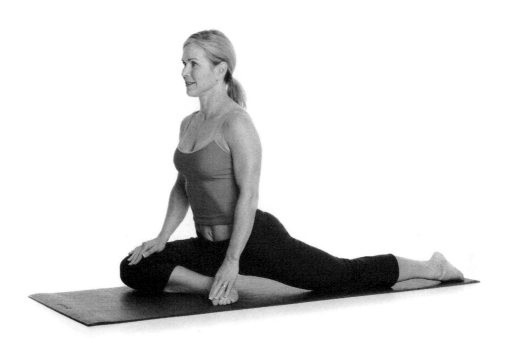

Kneel and then sit with your hips back on your heels. Lift your hips slightly and, keeping your right knee bent, stretch your left leg back to a half-split position. (You can rest your right thigh on the floor so your right foot is positioned in front of your left hip.) Place your left knee on the floor with the leg fully extended. Open your chest and lift your head to look toward the ceiling. Then release and switch legs.

CHILD'S POSE

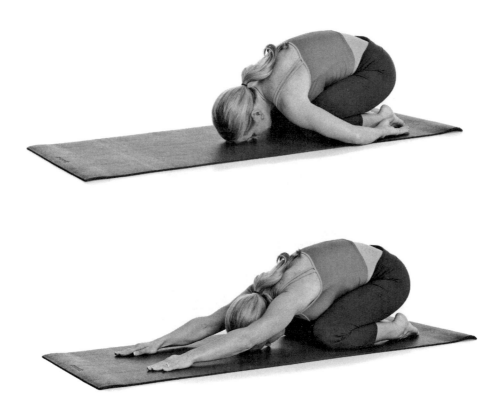

Kneel and then sit with your hips back on your heels. Lower your upper body down over your lap and rest your forehead on the floor. Rest your arms at your sides, palms facing up.

Or you can extend your arms straight out in front of you, reaching and spreading your fingers. Relax your neck, face, and shoulders as you take deep, slow breaths.

FLEXIBILITY LOG

Make photocopies of this log and use them to keep track of each and every one of the *Prevention*'s Shortcuts you take. Three to 5 days a week, you want to check off at least one flexibility workout. Check off one of the cardio walking workouts every day, and do a second one at least 3 days a week. Also remember to give yourself extra credit every time you squeeze in a 1-Minute Wonder, Lifestyle Shortcut, or *Prevention*'s Shortcut from other chapters.

	SUN	MON	TUES	WED	THU	FRI	SAT
Flexibility							
Workout A							
Workout B							
Workout C							
Cardio (see Chapter 4)							
Need for Speed							
Fast and Focused							
Strong and Steady							
Pyramid Power							
Rolling Hills							
Conquer the Mountain							
1-Minute Wonder							
Let Your Feet Do the Walking (page 36)							
Tap Your Toes! (page 76)							
Do "Invisible" Exercise (page 99)							
Multitasking Moves (page 149)							
Stealth Leg Slimmers (page 243)							

(continued)

	SUN	MON	TUES	WED	THU	FRI	SAT
Sneaky Arm Shapers (page 295)							
Armchair Athletics (page 328)							
Lifestyle Shortcut							
Walk This Way (page 77)							
Take It Outside! (page 80)							
Take Action! (page 144)							
Just Say No (page 178)							
Use Flower Power (page 179)							
Think Positive! (page 180)							
Get Sleep! (page 190)							
Drink Up! (page 191)							
Laugh It Up . . . and Off (page 297)							
Hit the Pound (page 299)							
Hoop It Up (page 329)							
Step Up to the Plate (page 358)							
Live for the Future (page 360)							
Other *Prevention*'s Shortcuts							

Notes (goals, feelings, etc.): _____
_____
_____
_____
_____
_____

TAKE A STAND

You know how stiff you feel sometimes in the morning after 6 to 8 hours of sleeping in the same position? That creakiness only goes away once you start moving, increase your circulation, and lubricate your joints with your body's natural synovial fluid. If you go from your bed to your minivan to your desk chair and spend 80 percent of your day with your hips bent in a seated position and your back hunched over a steering wheel or keyboard, guess what? That's the way your body is going to be inclined to stay, even when you try to stand up! That's especially true as we get older.

It's ironic, but kids are actually better designed to be sedentary than adults (who are forced to sit at a desk for hours on end!). Think of how a kid can sit perfectly still, twisted up like a pretzel while watching a movie or playing a board game, and pop up pain free as soon as the activity's done. You try that, and your back, knees, and hips will be screaming for mercy! As we age, it's imperative that we move our skeleton to stay mobile.

The simple act of standing is essential for maintaining flexibility. Every time you stand erect, you lengthen your spine, open your hips, and extend your hamstrings out of their normally shortened position. Thankfully, my job is active and keeps me moving, so I don't have to sit for too long. But my cowriter, Selene Yeager, is often stuck at her desk for hours on end. She swears by switching positions often and standing up at least once an hour to stretch her legs and take her eyes off the screen. "I use a drafting chair, so I can adjust the height periodically, which forces me to change my posture and sit a little differently," she says. "At home, I'll sit on an inflated exercise ball, which wakes up my posture muscles and forces me to sit straight. Or, when I can, I'll sit on the floor, so I can stretch my legs and hips while I read or work."

BUILD YOUR BONES

In case you need more incentive to get up out of your chair, the latest International Osteoporosis Foundation report reveals that women who sit for more than 9 hours a day are 50 percent more likely to break a hip than those who sit less than 6 hours a day. Sitting not only shortens your muscles and connective tissues but leads to

1-MINUTE WONDER
ARMCHAIR ATHLETICS

To keep rigor mortis from setting in when you're stuck in a seated position, sneak in some stretches. A number of great moves you can do without leaving your chair can stretch your glutes, hips, back, chest, and shoulders. Here are a few of my favorites. Hold each one for 15 to 30 seconds, stringing together a few to create a 1-Minute Wonder!

Sitting reach (stretches abs, chest, and shoulders). Sit in a chair, feet firmly planted, back straight. Extend your arms overhead, palms facing each other. Slowly arch your spine over the chair back as far as comfortably possible.

Chair reach and drop (stretches arms, back, and shoulders). Sit on the edge of a chair, feet firmly planted, back straight. Bring your arms up behind your back, hands clasped, and slowly lift them away from your back as far as comfortably possible. Lean forward from your hips, so that your chest touches your thighs, and continue lifting your arms toward the ceiling.

Seated figure 4 (stretches glutes, lower back, and hips). Sit in a chair with your legs bent and feet flat on the floor. Cross your right ankle over your left knee, so your calf is parallel to the floor and your right knee is pointing to the right. Keeping your back straight, lean forward from the hips until you feel a stretch deep in your right glute muscle. Repeat to each side.

De-slump stretch (stretches chest, shoulders, and upper back). Sit on the edge of a chair with your legs open and pelvis tilted slightly forward. Lift your chest and squeeze your shoulder blades together and down away from your ears. Extend your arms out from your body at 45-degree angles and reach them slightly behind you, palms facing forward.

Sit and twist (stretches back, shoulders, and sides). Sit up tall in a chair, feet flat on the floor. Place your right hand across your body onto your left upper arm. Reach your left arm across your chest, and immediately twist to the right and grasp the back of the chair with your left hand, bringing your chin over your right shoulder as you turn. Repeat to each side.

thinning of your bones, since they aren't at all challenged by gravity—the force that stimulates them to grow.

Brittle bones can lead to a collapse in the spine, leading to the humpbacked appearance some elderly women have and seriously limiting range of motion in the shoulders as well as the spine. Strength training is a great bone builder, as is any activity that has a little impact such as tennis, golf, or even just dribbling a basketball with your kids or grandkids and shooting hoops in the driveway. Remember, too, to get at least 1,000 mg of calcium (the amount in three glasses of milk) a day.

THE FOOD CONNECTION

What does food have to do with flexibility? Not a whole lot, unless what you eat is making you overweight. Excess weight can get in the way of your normal range of motion, limiting how far you can bend, reach, and twist. Weight also puts added stress and strain on your joints, increasing the wear and tear they have to endure and putting them at increased risk for degenerative diseases like osteoarthritis, which can make any movement painful.

LIFESTYLE SHORTCUT
HOOP IT UP

Sometimes child's play is the best thing for adult bodies. All those great kids' games like tag and kickball and playground fun take your body through a full range of motion while letting your mind relax and laugh. For flexibility in your back and hips, the most "therapeutic" kids' play may be with a hula hoop!

Swinging your hips to keep the hoop in motion rotates your vertebrae in a full range of motion they never see during everyday life (unless you moonlight as a belly dancer), and it's good exercise. You can even buy a weighted hoop called a Heavy Hoop. These foam-covered steel rings come in weights ranging from 1 to 7 pounds, and they make your abs and obliques work twice as hard as a lightweight hoop. Research shows that vigorous gyrating with a Heavy Hoop can fry up to 110 calories in just 10 minutes! Now that's no child's play.

The best part is, it takes *very* little weight loss to make a very big difference in the pressure you put on your joints. In fact, a new study shows that for each pound of body weight you lose, there is a 4-pound reduction in knee joint stress. Over just 1 mile, that adds up to more than 4,800 pounds of pressure! Lose 10 pounds and each knee is subjected to 48,000 fewer pounds of compressive load. By following the Clean-Eating Shortcuts rules along with one of the *Prevention*'s Shortcuts weight loss workouts, you can easily lose a pound a week and (literally) take a load off your knees and off your hips, ankles, and spine, too.

Finally, when you lose weight, your clothes will be looser—another flexibility booster. Clothes that bind your waist or constrict your hips and thighs—the places most of us carry excess pounds—make it nearly impossible to move through even a limited range of motion. (This is true for slim women, too. I'm sure we all remember the days when skin-tight "designer" jeans were all the rage, and millions of women couldn't even bend their hips properly to sit down!) Wear less-restrictive clothes that allow you to move freely when possible, and, if needed, work on reaching a healthy weight.

CHAPTER 13

Beat Back Pain

Line up 10 people in a room, and 8 of them will have a bout of back pain at some point in their lives. Back pain is the number one complaint doctors hear, and as people become heavier and more sedentary, it's becoming even more common. Decades ago, doctors ordered bed rest for back pain. Now the order of the day is to get up and move, even if it hurts, because too little activity can lead to loss of strength and flexibility and even more pain. UCLA researchers proved this point in a recent study of 600 chronic back pain sufferers. In a yearlong survey of their back pain episodes, they found that those who exercised regularly were 31 percent less likely to experience an increase in pain than their sedentary peers.

That's not to say you're immune to back pain just because you're slim and active. I know bike racers, runners, and otherwise healthy people of all ages who have been stricken with lower-back pain. But studies show that active folks who play weekend warrior are considerably more likely to suffer back pain injuries than those who do a little something every day (the heart and soul of the *Prevention*'s Shortcuts system). Most episodes of back pain clear up on their own, so the best long-term treatment for a healthy back is preventive medicine. That's why I included a special chapter on beating back pain in the *Prevention*'s Shortcuts system.

Lower-back pain is caused by many things, including weak back muscles, tight back and leg muscles, and, believe it or not, weak muscles in the belly. The *Prevention*'s Shortcuts system incorporates a combination of exercises that provide strengthening for the lower back and abdominals, as well as flexibility training for the lower back, hips, and legs.

LOSE YOUR BELLY, SAVE YOUR BACK

Imagine taking a 5-pound bag of sugar and tying it around your waist right at your navel. After 10 minutes, you'd feel like sitting down because your back hurt. Think about it! If you've ever been pregnant, you know *exactly* what I mean! In the final few weeks of my third pregnancy, just standing up out of a chair was stressful on my back. In effect, that's what it's like to carry extra weight around your belly. Belly fat pulls your lower spine forward, causing your back to arch, which compresses the disks and causes pain. As you shrink your waistline, your back straightens and your abdominals can better support your spine. Your posture improves and your back pain diminishes.

A healthy diet not only helps you lose weight, which soothes your spine, but also can keep your vertebrae strong by helping you build bone. The key is getting plenty of calcium (at least 1,000 mg a day) and vitamin D (400 IUs a day). Most adults don't get enough of either. Sunshine is your best source of vitamin D. So make a point to go outside and expose your face, arms, and hands to the sun for 5 minutes a day. (If you're going to be out in the sun any longer, you'll need to wear sunscreen. A little sun is healthy; too much, as you already know, is not.) Calcium-rich foods include leafy green vegetables, fortified foods like orange juice, and dairy products like low-fat yogurt and skim milk.

To shed your spare tire, you also need exercise—and plenty of it. By turning up the intensity of your workouts, you can burn belly fat even faster, according to a Duke University study of 175 overweight men and women. To test the waist-whittling effects of higher-intensity exercise, the researchers had one-third of the volunteers stroll leisurely for 30 minutes a day, 5 days a week; another one-third jog or walk very briskly for the same amount of time; and the final one-third stay sedentary. After 8 months, the couch potatoes actually got heavier. Worse, their levels of dangerous belly fat increased by a whopping 8.6 percent! The easy exercisers kept their waistlines from widening, but they actually did gain a little weight (about 1½ pounds). Far and away, the group that reaped the greatest rewards were the high-intensity exercisers. They not only lost 6 pounds but also shrank both their waistlines and levels of organ-smothering abdominal fat by 7 percent. How hard did they have to work? A 6 to 8 on an RPE scale of 1 to 10—about the intensity of a brisk uphill walk or pedaling a bike 12 mph. Good news: That's the exact intensity of *Prevention*'s Shortcuts cardio workouts in Chapter 4.

SPINE SMARTS

Being strong and active doesn't give you license to abuse your back. To keep pain at bay, you need to exercise some healthy habits as well as your muscles. Following these basic back safety tips will help save your spine.

Lift with your legs. The vast majority of lower-back injuries happen when you bend and twist from the waist. The disks in your spine are cushioned by a liquid gel and surrounded by a ring of cartilage, not unlike a jelly doughnut. As you bend forward from the waist, you push the gel toward the back and stress the cartilage. When you twist from that position, the cartilage can tear, allowing the gel to bulge out and cause pain. Whether you're picking up a 15-pound dumbbell or a pair of socks, bend from the hips and knees and lift with your legs. If you're lifting something heavy, like a 40-pound toddler, "brace" yourself before you lift. Pull your abs in tight and bear down to stabilize your spine, then bend and lift with your legs. Keep the weight as close to your body as possible as you carry it, to reduce stress on your spine.

Practice your posture. Good posture protects your back. When you stand with your joints in proper alignment, there is minimal stress on your supporting muscles and less tension on the ligaments holding the joints of your spine together. Poor posture can be a hard habit to break, especially if you've always stood or sat with a slouch or a slump. But with practice, you can make sitting and standing straight second nature. Here's how your reflection should look in the mirror.

> Your head should be straight up with your chin level to the floor; your earlobes should fall directly in line with the center of your shoulders.
>
> Shoulder blades should be back and down, and your breastbone lifted so your chest is open.
>
> Hips should be facing squarely forward, and your knees should point straight ahead.
>
> Hold your abs tight and keep your pelvis neutral. Your tailbone shouldn't be tilted forward or back.

Your sitting posture should be very similar.

> Your back should be straight, with shoulders back. Your butt should touch the back of the chair, and your weight should be evenly distributed on both hips.

Avoid standing or sitting frozen in the exact same position for too long. Lift a leg. Get up and stretch. Even if you have good posture, your body needs a chance to move and loosen.

Sleep well. You (I hope) sleep 7 to 8 hours a night, so your sleep posture is extremely important for back health. Experts say the most spine-friendly positions are on your back with a bedroll or pillow tucked under your knees, or on your side with your knees slightly bent (put a small pillow between your knees for added comfort). Avoid sleeping flat on your back or belly. Both of those positions place stress on your spine.

The following workouts will strengthen and stretch your spine-supporting muscles in just 2 weeks. If you have back pain right now, it's a good idea to clear your exercise program with your doctor. Otherwise, you can do these workouts every day. For optimum results, aim to do at least three workouts a week. As always, for total-body wellness, you should also do at least one of the Chapter 4 cardio workouts every day plus a second one of those workouts 3 to 5 days a week.

And whenever possible, try a Lifestyle Shortcut, a 1-Minute Wonder, or any of the *Prevention*'s Shortcuts workouts from any other chapters in the book that strike you as fun and interesting. Use the log on page 356 to keep track of what you've done each day.

WORKOUT A

Hold each pose for about 40 seconds. Do 12 to 15 reps (on both right and left sides, where appropriate) of each exercise. Complete the whole workout twice.

Cat/Cow

Spinal Balance and Crunch

Swimming

Seated Butterfly

Child's Pose

Pilates Crunch

CAT/COW

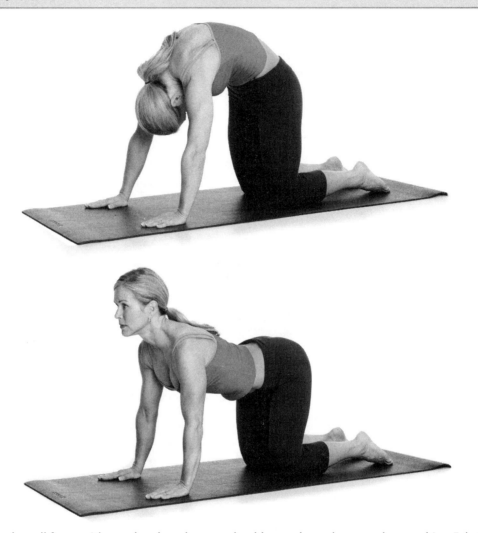

Kneel on all fours, with your hands under your shoulders and your knees under your hips. Exhale and tuck your tailbone under, round your spine, and drop your head as though you are looking for your navel. Push evenly through your hands and knees, and arch your upper back toward the sky.

Continue from Cat into Cow (back extension): Extend your spine, lift your tailbone toward the sky, and drop your belly down toward the floor. Look up. Try to lengthen the crown of your head away from your tailbone.

SPINAL BALANCE AND CRUNCH

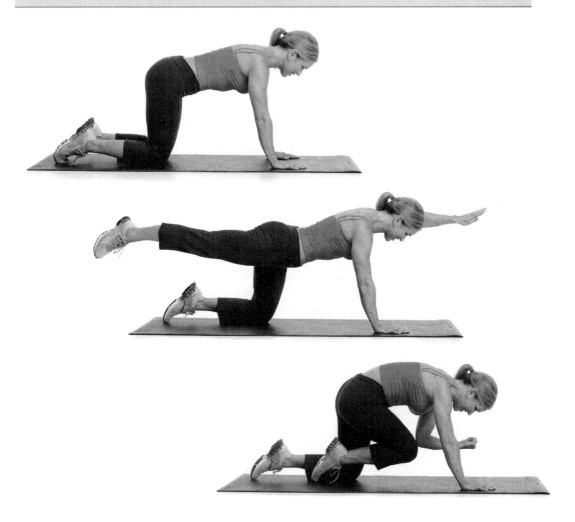

Kneel on all fours, with your hands directly beneath your shoulders and your knees directly beneath your hips. Keep your back straight and your head in line with your spine.

Draw your navel toward your spine and simultaneously raise your left arm and right leg, extending them in line with your back so your fingers are pointing straight ahead and your toes are pointing back. Hold for 2 seconds.

Then contract your abs and draw your left elbow and your right knee together, beneath your torso. Complete a full set, then switch sides.

SWIMMING

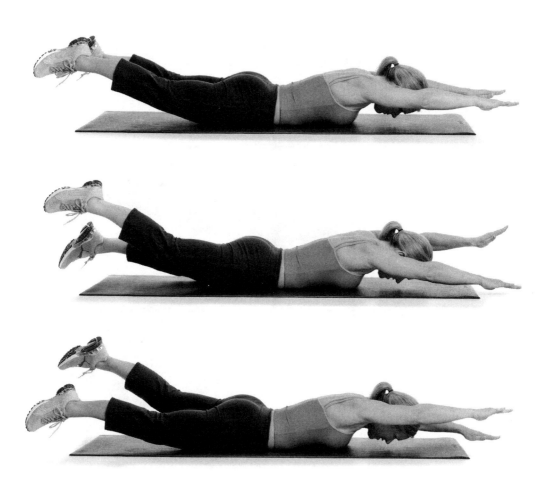

Lie facedown on the floor with your arms extended out in front of you and your legs extended back. Lift your limbs up off the ground and keep your abs tight. Point your fingertips and toes to create a long spine.

Flutter opposite arms and legs simultaneously, while breathing smoothly and steadily.

SEATED BUTTERFLY

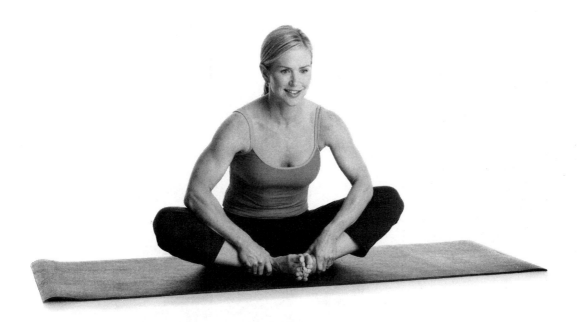

Begin in a seated position with the soles of your feet together. Place your hands on your ankles and press your elbows into your inner thighs. Gently push your knees toward the floor. Press your sitting bones down against the floor and lengthen your spine, reaching toward the sky with the crown of your head. Drop your shoulders away from your ears and gently tuck in your chin. Inhale and exhale a little farther into the stretch.

CHILD'S POSE

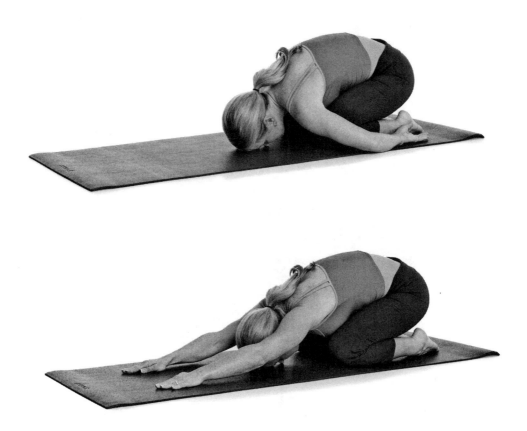

Kneel and then sit with your hips back on your heels. Lower your upper body down over your lap and rest your forehead on the floor. Rest your arms at your sides, palms facing up.

Or you can extend your arms straight out in front of you, reaching and spreading your fingers. Relax your neck, face, and shoulders as you take deep, slow breaths.

PILATES CRUNCH

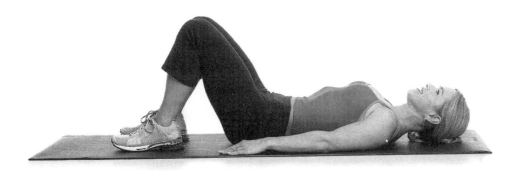

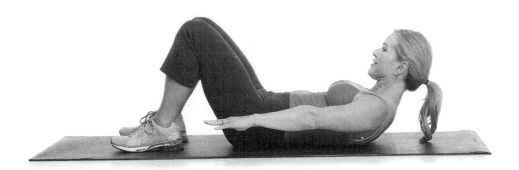

Lie faceup on the floor with your knees bent, your feet hip-width apart and flat on the ground, and your arms at your sides, palms on the floor.

Visualize sliding your rib cage to your pelvis as you pull your navel toward your spine, contract your abs, and sequentially roll your head, shoulders, and upper back off the floor. As you perform the move, lengthen through the back of your neck and tuck your chin slightly toward your chest, while keeping your arms parallel to the floor. Lower back to the starting position. This is the difference between mindlessly crunching and really pulling in and activating your deep transversus abdominis to make your core muscles work.

WORKOUT B

Hold each pose for about 40 seconds. Do 12 to 15 reps (on both right and left sides, where appropriate) of each exercise. Complete the whole workout twice.

Seated Butterfly

Half Roll-Back

Full-Body Roll-Up

Seated Spinal Twist

Side Hip Lift

Pigeon

SEATED BUTTERFLY

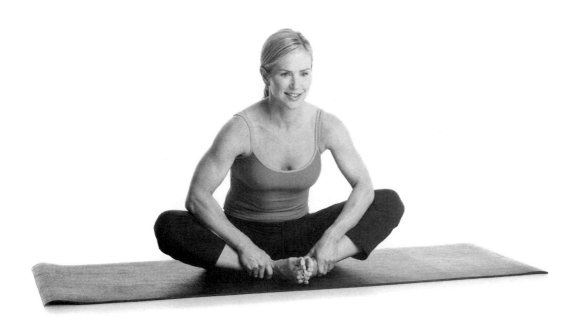

Begin in a seated position with the soles of your feet together. Place your hands on your ankles and press your elbows into your inner thighs. Gently push your knees toward the floor. Press your sitting bones down against the floor and lengthen your spine, reaching toward the sky with the crown of your head. Drop your shoulders away from your ears and gently tuck in your chin. Inhale and exhale a little farther into the stretch.

HALF ROLL-BACK

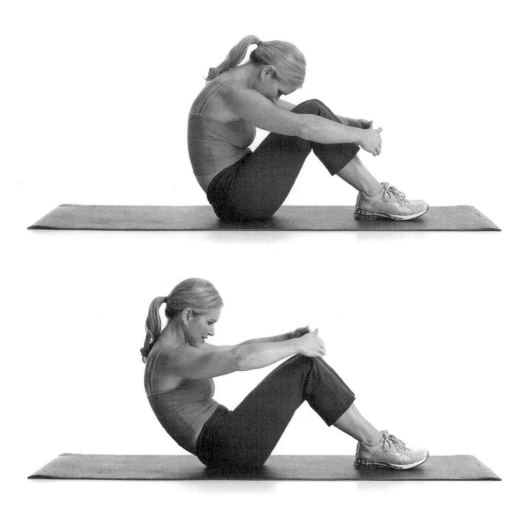

Sit on the floor with your knees bent and your feet and knees separated slightly. Pull your navel toward your spine and curl your spine forward so your torso is bent over your legs in a C shape. Reach your arms forward, with your shoulders relaxed.

Exhale and, maintaining a C shape with your spine, roll halfway back by tucking your tailbone and lowering vertebrae by vertebrae. Inhale and pull your abs even closer toward your spine. Then exhale and contract your abs to return to the starting position. Maintain a rounded spine throughout the movement.

FULL-BODY ROLL-UP

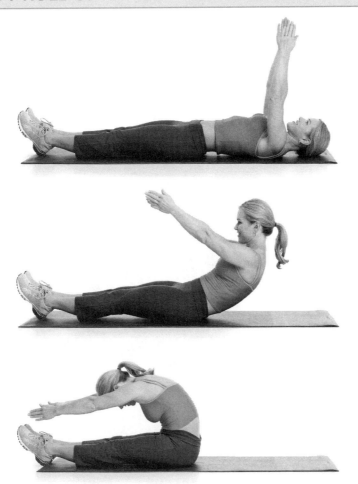

Lie faceup on the floor with your arms relaxed and extended straight up. Pull your navel toward your spine to engage your abdominal muscles as you inhale and stretch your arms upward.

Exhale, lengthen the back of your neck, tuck your chin toward your chest, and, keeping your navel pulled toward your spine, curl forward with your arms extending in front of you. Visualize leading with the top of your head to create a C curve, curling forward until you are reaching for your toes. Inhale as you stay rounded.

Begin reversing direction, uncurling your body. Exhale as you continue to "drip" your spine back to the floor, one vertebrae at a time, slowly lowering back to the starting position.

SEATED SPINAL TWIST

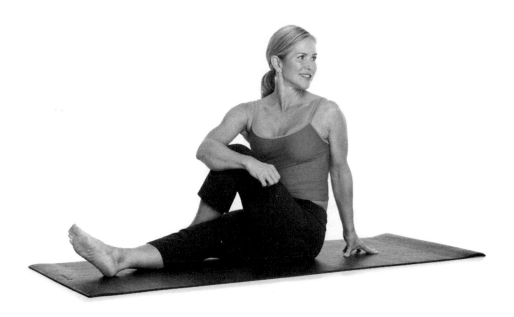

Sit on the floor with your legs extended. Place your hands on the floor behind your back for support. Cross your left leg over the right and place your left foot on the floor on the outside of your right knee. Keeping your spine long and tall, twist your torso toward the left, wrapping your right arm around your left knee. Look over your left shoulder. Hold. Then switch sides.

SIDE HIP LIFT

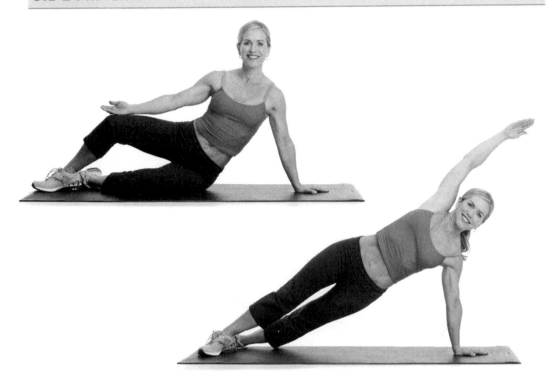

Sit on your left hip with your legs extended to your right, knees slightly bent. Cross your right foot just in front of your left. Place your left hand on the floor, in line with your left shoulder, for support. Extend your right arm and place your right hand on your right knee, palm facing up.

Pull your navel toward your spine, contract your obliques, and lift your hips off the floor while extending your right arm overhead, so your body forms a straight diagonal line. Then, without bending your left arm, lower your hips and right arm back to the starting position.

Complete a set, then repeat on your other side.

If you're a beginner, keep your left knee on the floor.

PIGEON

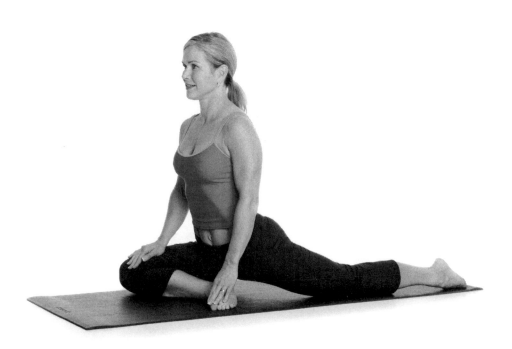

Kneel and then sit with your hips back on your heels. Lift your hips slightly and, keeping your right knee bent, stretch your left leg back to a half-split position. (You can rest your right thigh on the floor so your right foot is positioned in front of your left hip.) Place your left knee on the floor with the leg fully extended. Open your chest and lift your head to look toward the ceiling. Then release and switch legs.

WORKOUT C

Hold each pose for about 40 seconds. Do 12 to 15 reps (on both right and left sides, where appropriate) of each exercise. Complete the whole workout twice.

Cat/Cow

Bridge "Bun" Lift

Half Roll-Back

Child's Pose

Straight-Leg Reverse Curl

Pigeon

CAT/COW

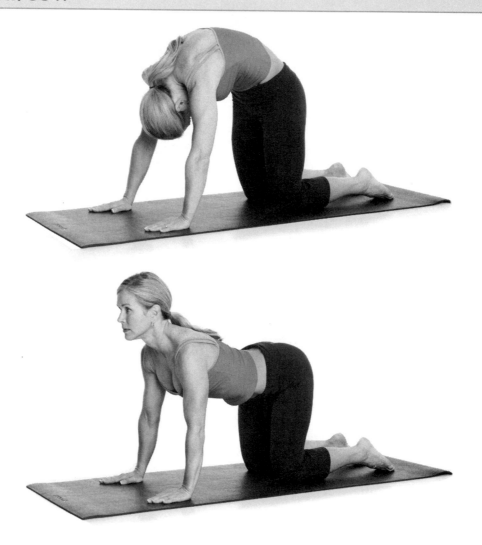

Kneel on all fours, with your hands under your shoulders and your knees under your hips. Exhale and tuck your tailbone under, round your spine, and drop your head as though you are looking for your navel. Push evenly through your hands and knees, and arch your upper back toward the sky.

Continue from Cat into Cow (back extension): Extend your spine, lift your tailbone toward the sky, and drop your belly down toward the floor. Look up. Try to lengthen the crown of your head away from your tailbone.

BRIDGE "BUN" LIFT

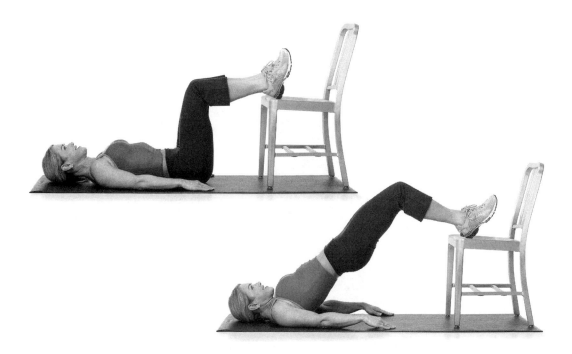

Lie on the floor and place your heels hip-width apart on the edge of a chair seat (or on a step, if a chair is too high), arms down by your sides, palms down.

Keeping your hips square to the ceiling and your navel pulled toward your spine, press into your heels, squeeze your buns, and lift your hips toward the ceiling so your body forms a straight line from your knees to your shoulders. You can use your hands for balance but not to push yourself up. Lower back to the starting position.

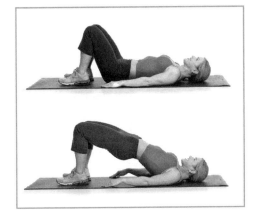

Beginners can try this first without a chair, feet on the floor.

HALF ROLL-BACK

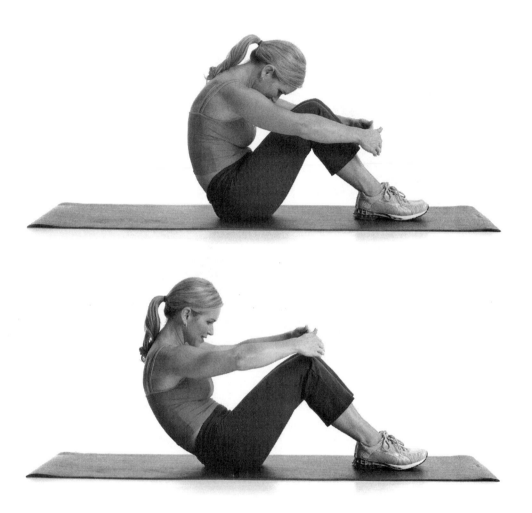

Sit on the floor with your knees bent and your feet and knees separated slightly. Pull your navel toward your spine and curl your spine forward so your torso is bent over your legs in a C shape. Reach your arms forward, with your shoulders relaxed.

Exhale and, maintaining a C shape with your spine, roll halfway back by tucking your tailbone and lowering vertebrae by vertebrae. Inhale and pull your abs even closer toward your spine. Then exhale and contract your abs to return to the starting position. Maintain a rounded spine throughout the movement.

CHILD'S POSE

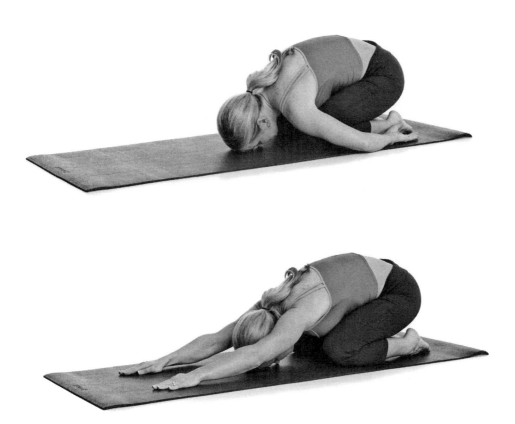

Kneel and then sit with your hips back on your heels. Lower your upper body down over your lap and rest your forehead on the floor. Rest your arms at your sides, palms facing up.

Or you can extend your arms straight out in front of you, reaching and spreading your fingers. Relax your neck, face, and shoulders as you take deep, slow breaths.

STRAIGHT-LEG REVERSE CURL

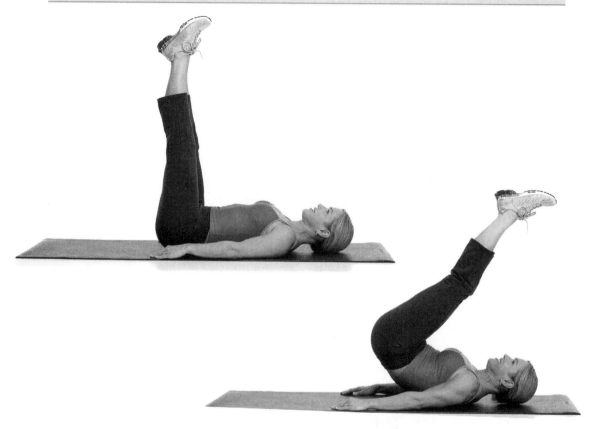

Lie faceup on the floor with your arms at your sides, legs extended into the air at a 90-degree angle to your tailbone on the mat.

Draw your navel toward your spine to scoop your abs and curl your hips off the floor so your feet move slightly over your head. Hold for a moment, then slowly lower back to the starting position.

If your hamstrings are tight, keep your knees slightly bent throughout this exercise.

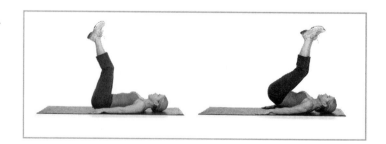

PIGEON

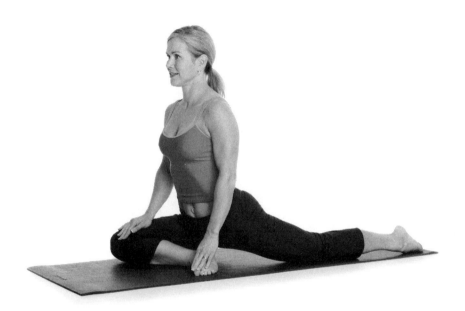

Kneel and then sit with your hips back on your heels. Lift your hips slightly and, keeping your right knee bent, stretch your left leg back to a half-split position. (You can rest your right thigh on the floor so your right foot is positioned in front of your left hip.) Place your left knee on the floor with the leg fully extended. Open your chest and lift your head to look toward the ceiling. Then release and switch legs.

BEAT BACK PAIN LOG

Make photocopies of this log and use them to keep track of each and every one of the *Prevention*'s Shortcuts you take. Three to 5 days a week, you want to check off at least one back workout. Check off one of the cardio walking workouts every day, and do a second one at least 3 days a week. Also remember to give yourself extra credit every time you squeeze in a 1-Minute Wonder, Lifestyle Shortcut, or *Prevention*'s Shortcut from other chapters.

	SUN	MON	TUES	WED	THU	FRI	SAT
Beat Back Pain							
Workout A							
Workout B							
Workout C							
Cardio (see Chapter 4)							
Need for Speed							
Fast and Focused							
Strong and Steady							
Pyramid Power							
Rolling Hills							
Conquer the Mountain							
1-Minute Wonder							
Let Your Feet Do the Walking (page 36)							
Tap Your Toes! (page 76)							
Do "Invisible" Exercise (page 99)							
Multitasking Moves (page 149)							
Stealth Leg Slimmers (page 243)							
Sneaky Arm Shapers (page 295)							

	SUN	MON	TUES	WED	THU	FRI	SAT
Armchair Athletics (page 328)							
Lifestyle Shortcut							
Walk This Way (page 77)							
Take It Outside! (page 80)							
Take Action! (page 144)							
Just Say No (page 178)							
Use Flower Power (page 179)							
Think Positive! (page 180)							
Get Sleep! (page 190)							
Drink Up! (page 191)							
Laugh It Up . . . and Off (page 297)							
Hit the Pound (page 299)							
Hoop It Up (page 329)							
Step Up to the Plate (page 358)							
Live for the Future (page 360)							
Other *Prevention*'s Shortcuts							

Notes (goals, feelings, etc.): _____

_____

_____

_____

_____

_____

_____

HAVE A BALL!

If you buy one piece of workout equipment (aside from your hand weights, of course), make it a stability or exercise ball. My clients with back pain issues *love* these large, lightweight, inflatable balls for stretching out. Just lying back on one feels *so* great. They also make ab exercises like crunches more challenging because when you lie back on a stability ball, your abdominals are extended farther than when you are lying on the floor.

Inflatable exercise balls are available at all major sporting goods stores as well as department stores like Target. Be sure to pick one that's the right size for you. If you're under 5 feet 1 inch, choose a 45-centimeter ball. A 55-centimeter ball will fit women between 5 feet 1 inch and 5 feet 6 inches. Go for 65 centimeters if you're 5 feet 7 inches to 5 feet 11 inches and 75 centimeters if you're taller than that.

LIFESTYLE SHORTCUT
STEP UP TO THE PLATE

One of the most effective weight loss devices ever invented is sitting right in your kitchen. In fact, you probably have a lot them. They're called plates, and eating off them can help you cut dozens, if not hundreds, of calories every day. It works like this: Instead of opening the fridge, popping open a plastic leftovers container, and mindlessly scooping food into your mouth, you put the amount you want to eat on the plate and eat it. Sitting down at the table is a bonus, but you don't even have to go that far.

Some of the healthiest, consistently slim women I know make it a rule to never eat out of containers, whether they're potato chip bags, Chinese takeout cartons, or milk jugs. Putting food on a plate and a beverage in a glass is the only way to see (and control) how much you're eating. And while it's a cinch to polish off the brownie pan, pinch by pinch, you would never eat a whole plateful. Even better, use the salad plates. In today's oversize dish world, they're plenty big enough to hold a whole meal.

Conclusion

Congratulations! You now have the tools to move forward and be successful. Knowledge is power, and with the *Prevention*'s Shortcuts system, you have the power to be self-confident by knowing what to do without needing lots of time. Self-confident people face their fears, learn from their mistakes, forgive themselves, and keep moving forward positively. Very often, they have no more talent or capabilities than anyone else, just the confidence to do it till it works!

This program is a two-way street: You have me and the women who shared their *Prevention*'s Shortcuts Success Stories for motivation and my workouts as a tool—but you have to do the work. Whenever you feel a surge of motivation, ride it like a wave. Follow my three Cs: commitment, convenience, and consistency. All the studies in this book prove that being consistent far outweighs the results of the all-or-nothing attitude.

I am so hopeful for you and confident that you will become a great success, like so many women I've watched transform before my very eyes! I look forward to hearing from you on your journey. I have learned so much about women and exercise during the past 20 years, and I'm absolutely a believer that everyone has a chance at creating a healthy lifestyle. I can't promise you there won't be roadblocks along the way. In fact, I can guarantee there will be! One of the life lessons I drill into my kids' heads is "Life is not fair." Believe me, I have had my knocks of hard luck, but something inside me always keeps me moving in a positive direction. Remember this: "Genetics loads your gun, but environment pulls your trigger." It's what you eat, what you do, and the choices you make that shape your life!

I'm your biggest fan right now, so get moving! When colleagues say to me, "Chris, you make it too simple," I say, "Exactly, and that's why my clients are losing weight and feeling great!" In our overstimulated, overbooked, and overstressed world, it's nice to know that a little effort still goes a long way.

I know you can do it, and I'd love to hear about your success. Keep me informed or ask me any questions you might have by e-mailing me from www.ChrisFreytag. com. Just click on Contact at the top of the Web page and fill in the e-mail form. I'll always get back to you.

Stay healthy!

Chris Freytag

LIFESTYLE SHORTCUT
LIVE FOR THE FUTURE

It's easy to get mad at your old self. Many of my clients bemoan the past. "If only I hadn't let myself go, this wouldn't be so hard now." "If only I had known ..." "If only ...," "if only ...," "if only ..." The past is gone. If you're beating yourself up over it, you've learned from it, so it's time to put it down, pick up the present, and look forward to the future. Besides, a recent health and fitness study shows that what you did when you were young counts much less than what you're doing right now.

When researchers reviewed past and recent activity levels of more than 5,000 men and women, they found that those who were physically active at the time of the survey were 40 percent less likely to die during the 16-year follow-up than those who were mostly sedentary, regardless of how active they were in the past. There's no time like the present to start living the life you wish you'd lived before. It's like Abe Lincoln famously said, "Most folks are about as happy as they make up their minds to be!" I always tell my clients, "I sympathize with you, but I don't feel sorry for you." I am always willing to lend an ear. But I won't let you dig yourself into a deep hole. Climb out and keep going!

Index

Boldface page references indicate photographs. <u>Underscored</u> references indicate boxed text.

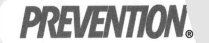

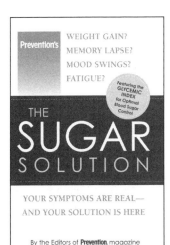

Prevention®'s The Sugar Solution

by the editors of *Prevention*® magazine with Ann Fittante, MS, RD

In addition to diabetes, blood-sugar imbalance can set the stage for a host of health problems—from unexplained weight gain, fatigue, and poor concentration to heart disease and stroke. This national bestseller is an easy-to-follow, drug-free program that can bring blood sugar into balance in just one month.

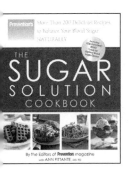

Prevention®'s The Sugar Solution Cookbook

by the editors of *Prevention*® magazine with Ann Fittante, MD, RD

This follow-up to *The Sugar Solution* offers more than 200 delicious recipes that stabilize blood sugar, which is the key to losing weight quickly, safely, and permanently.

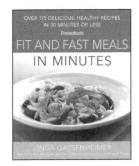

Prevention®'s Fit and Fast Meals in Minutes

by Linda Gassenheimer

Quick, healthy, great-tasting meals by the author of the enormously popular, nationally syndicated "Dinner in Minutes" newspaper column.

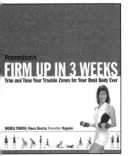

Prevention®'s Firm Up in 3 Weeks

by Michele Stanten

From *Prevention*® magazine's fitness expert, a personalized daily workout and walking program that firms up arms, abs, butt, and thighs in just three short weeks.

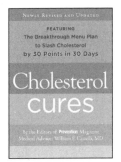

Cholesterol Cures

by the editors of *Prevention*® health books

This updated edition presents hundreds of all-natural solutions to high cholesterol, featuring the breakthrough menu plan to slash cholesterol 30 points in 30 days.

Available in stores everywhere!

Don't miss the DVD companion to *Shortcuts to Big Weight Loss* and more great Chris Freytag titles!

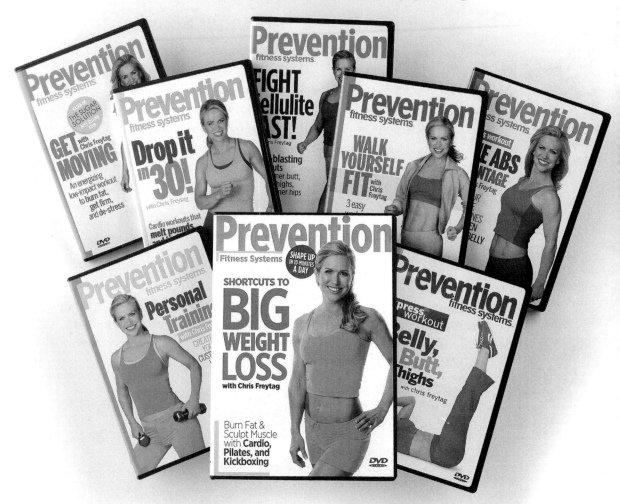

No matter what your goal, from building better cardiovascular health to shedding excess pounds, odds are Chris Freytag has an easy-to-follow DVD to help you achieve it.

And since each has been designed by the fitness editors of *Prevention* magazine, you know that they're safe, effective, and made with your total health in mind.

AVAILABLE IN STORES NOW!
www.prevention.com/shop

200846101